T0214050

# Lecture Notes of the Institute for Computer Sciences, Social Informatics and Telecommunications Engineering 360

Editorial Board Members

Ozgur Akan
   *Middle East Technical University, Ankara, Turkey*
Paolo Bellavista
   *University of Bologna, Bologna, Italy*
Jiannong Cao
   *Hong Kong Polytechnic University, Hong Kong, China*
Geoffrey Coulson
   *Lancaster University, Lancaster, UK*
Falko Dressler
   *University of Erlangen, Erlangen, Germany*
Domenico Ferrari
   *Università Cattolica Piacenza, Piacenza, Italy*
Mario Gerla
   *UCLA, Los Angeles, USA*
Hisashi Kobayashi
   *Princeton University, Princeton, USA*
Sergio Palazzo
   *University of Catania, Catania, Italy*
Sartaj Sahni
   *University of Florida, Gainesville, USA*
Xuemin (Sherman) Shen ⓘ
   *University of Waterloo, Waterloo, Canada*
Mircea Stan
   *University of Virginia, Charlottesville, USA*
Xiaohua Jia
   *City University of Hong Kong, Kowloon, Hong Kong*
Albert Y. Zomaya
   *University of Sydney, Sydney, Australia*

More information about this series at http://www.springer.com/series/8197

Rossitza Goleva · Nuno Ricardo da Cruz Garcia ·
Ivan Miguel Pires (Eds.)

# IoT Technologies
# for HealthCare

7th EAI International Conference, HealthyIoT 2020
Viana do Castelo, Portugal, December 3, 2020
Proceedings

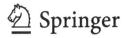 Springer

*Editors*
Rossitza Goleva 🆔
Informatics
New Bulgarian University
Sofia, Bulgaria

Nuno Ricardo da Cruz Garcia 🆔
University of Lisboa
Lisboa, Portugal

Ivan Miguel Pires 🆔
University of Beira Interior
Covilhã, Portugal

ISSN 1867-8211 ISSN 1867-822X (electronic)
Lecture Notes of the Institute for Computer Sciences, Social Informatics
and Telecommunications Engineering
ISBN 978-3-030-69962-8 ISBN 978-3-030-69963-5 (eBook)
https://doi.org/10.1007/978-3-030-69963-5

© ICST Institute for Computer Sciences, Social Informatics and Telecommunications Engineering 2021
This work is subject to copyright. All rights are reserved by the Publisher, whether the whole or part of the material is concerned, specifically the rights of translation, reprinting, reuse of illustrations, recitation, broadcasting, reproduction on microfilms or in any other physical way, and transmission or information storage and retrieval, electronic adaptation, computer software, or by similar or dissimilar methodology now known or hereafter developed.
The use of general descriptive names, registered names, trademarks, service marks, etc. in this publication does not imply, even in the absence of a specific statement, that such names are exempt from the relevant protective laws and regulations and therefore free for general use.
The publisher, the authors and the editors are safe to assume that the advice and information in this book are believed to be true and accurate at the date of publication. Neither the publisher nor the authors or the editors give a warranty, expressed or implied, with respect to the material contained herein or for any errors or omissions that may have been made. The publisher remains neutral with regard to jurisdictional claims in published maps and institutional affiliations.

This Springer imprint is published by the registered company Springer Nature Switzerland AG
The registered company address is: Gewerbestrasse 11, 6330 Cham, Switzerland

# Preface

Healthy IoT 2020, the 7th EAI International Conference on IoT Technologies for HealthCare, was planned to take place in Viana do Castelo, Portugal on 2 December, 2020 under the umbrella of the 6th annual SmartCity 360°Summit. However, due to the COVID-19 crises it was organized online on 3 Dec. 2020. The event was endorsed by the European Alliance for Innovation, an international professional community-based organization devoted to the advancement of innovation in the field of ICT.

Healthy IoT 2020 was the seventh edition of an international scientific event series dedicated to the Internet of Things and Healthcare. The Internet of Things together with cloud computing have evolved multiple existing and emerging technologies, solutions and services, and can provide heterogeneous approaches towards the delivery of Healthcare 4.0 to the broad range of citizens. Healthy IoT brings together technology experts, researchers, industry and international authorities contributing towards the design, development and deployment of healthcare solutions based on IoT technologies, standards and procedures.

The technical program of Healthy IoT 2020 consisted of 12 full papers in oral presentation sessions at the main workshop tracks. The papers submitted and presented during the workshop cover many health sensors and systems technologies, applications and services as well as solutions. Multiple topics have been covered, including: remote sensing of women during pregnancy with attention to drug addiction and emergency situations; noninvasive screening of the hearing of adults based on a smartphone application; use of pressure sensors on the insoles for activity and moving problem detection; continuous stress detection based on sensor information; classification of psychological conditions; analyses of the psychological response to acoustic stimuli using sensors; visual acuity analyses supported by wearable devices; early diagnosis of kidney problems using data mining classification; study of teenager's health at school with attention to physical activity; a proposal of scenarios and time scheduling for medical applications; development of wearable devices for sport and rehabilitation tracking; the security of remote medication processes.

Mladen Veinović organized a panel discussion on the role of IT and IoT in responding to epidemic/pandemic-related challenges. It turns out that IT plays a fundamental role in mitigating risks and consequences, and providing alternative ways of performing fundamental tasks.

Coordination with the steering chair, Imrich Chlamtac, as well as the valuable support of Aleksandar Jevremović, Susanna Spinsante, Bruno Silva, Nuno M. Garcia, Nuno Pombo, Mlađan Jovanović, Francisco Floréz-Revuelta, Luis Oliveira, Hugo Silva, Nenad Ristić, Marko Šarac and, Leonice Pereira were essential for the success of the workshop. We sincerely appreciate their continuous work and support.

We strongly believe that the Healthy IoT 2020 workshop provided a good forum for all researchers, developers and practitioners to discuss all scientific and technological aspects that are relevant to smart health. We also expect that the future Healthy IoT

2021 workshop will be as successful and stimulating, as indicated by the contributions presented in this volume.

December 2020

Aleksandar Jevremovic

Susanna Spinsante

Bruno Silva

Nuno M. Garcia

Nuno Pombo

Mladjan Jovanovic

Francisco Florez-Revuelta

Luis Oliveira

Hugo Silva

Nenad Ristic

Marko Sarac

Leonice Pereira

# Conference Organization

## Steering Committee

Imrich Chlamtac — Bruno Kessler Professor, University of Trento, Italy

## Organizing Committee

### General Chair

Aleksandar Jevremović — Singidunum University, Serbia

### General Co-chairs

Susanna Spinsante — Marche Polytechnic University, Italy
Bruno Silva — IADE-Universidade Europeia and Universidade da Beira Interior, Portugal

### TPC Chair and Co-chairs

Nuno Pombo — University of Beira Interior, Portugal
Mlađan Jovanović — Singidunum University, Serbia

### Sponsorship and Exhibit Chair

Leonice Pereira — University of Beira Interior, Portugal

### Local Chair

Luis Oliveira — Tomar Technology School, Portugal

### Workshops Chair

Francisco Floréz-Revuelta — University of Alicante, Spain

### Publicity and Social Media Chair

Hugo Silva — Instituto de Telecomunicações, Portugal

### Publications Chair

Rossitza Goleva — New Bulgarian University, Bulgaria

### Web Chairs

Nenad Ristić — Sinergija University, Bosnia and Herzegovina
Marko Šarac — Singidunum University, Serbia

**Posters and PhD Track Chair**

Nuno M. Garcia                  Universidade da Beira Interior, Portugal

**Panels Chair**

Mladen Veinović                 Singidunum University, Serbia

**Demos Chair**

Leonice Pereira                 University of Beira Interior, Portugal

## Technical Program Committee

| | |
|---|---|
| Alessia Paglialonga | Institute of Electronics, Computer and Telecommunication Engineering, Italy |
| An Braeken | Vrije Universiteit Brussel, Belgium |
| Andrii Shalaginov | Norwegian University of Science and Technology, Norway |
| Ciprian Dobre | National Institute for Research & Development in Informatics, Romania |
| Constandinos X. Mavromoustakis | University of Nicosia, Cyprus |
| Eftim Zdravevski | Saints Cyril and Methodius University, Macedonia |
| Ennio Gambi | Marche Polytechnic University, Italy |
| Emmanuel Conchon | University of Limoges, France |
| Henriques Zacarias | University of Beira Interior, Portugal |
| Ivan Ganchev | University of Limerick, Ireland, University of Plovdiv "Paisii Hilendarski", Bulgaria |
| Javier Medina Quero | University of Jaén, Spain |
| Lina Xu | University College Dublin, Ireland |
| Marko Šarac | Singidunum University, Serbia |
| Pedro Brandão | University of Porto, Portugal |
| Petre Lameski | Saints Cyril and Methodius University, Macedonia |
| Sandeep Pirbhulal | Norwegian University of Science and Technology, Norway |
| Saša Adamović | Singidunum University, Serbia |
| Stefania Costantini | University of L'Aquila (UNIVAQ), Italy |
| Virginie Felizardo | University of Beira Interior, Portugal |

# Contents

**Physical Data Tracking Wearables, Applications and Systems**

Development and Evaluation of a Novel Method for Adult Hearing
Screening: Towards a Dedicated Smartphone App. . . . . . . . . . . . . . . . . . 3
    *Edoardo Maria Polo, Marco Zanet, Marta Lenatti,*
    *Toon van Waterschoot, Riccardo Barbieri, and Alessia Paglialonga*

A Non-invasive Cloud-Based IoT System and Data Analytics Support
for Women Struggling with Drug Addictions During Pregnancy . . . . . . . . . 20
    *Victor Balogun, Oluwafemi A. Sarumi, and Oludolapo D. Balogun*

Sensors Characterization for a Calibration-Free Connected Smart Insole
for Healthy Ageing . . . . . . . . . . . . . . . . . . . . . . . . . . . . . . . . . . . . . 35
    *Luca Gioacchini, Angelica Poli, Stefania Cecchi, and Susanna Spinsante*

Novel Wearable System for Surface EMG Using Compact Electronic Board
and Printed Matrix of Electrodes. . . . . . . . . . . . . . . . . . . . . . . . . . . . . 55
    *Tiziano Fapanni, Nicola Francesco Lopomo, Emilio Sardini,*
    *and Mauro Serpelloni*

Chronic Kidney Disease Early Diagnosis Enhancing by Using Data Mining
Classification and Features Selection . . . . . . . . . . . . . . . . . . . . . . . . . . 61
    *Pedro A. Moreno-Sanchez*

Interpreting the Visual Acuity of the Human Eye with Wearable EEG
Device and SSVEP . . . . . . . . . . . . . . . . . . . . . . . . . . . . . . . . . . . . . 77
    *Danson Evan Garcia, Yi Liu , Kai Wen Zheng, Yi (Summer) Tao,*
    *Phillip V. Do, Cayden Pierce, and Steve Mann*

**Psychological Data Tracking Wearables, Applications and Systems**

Stress Detection with Deep Learning Approaches Using
Physiological Signals. . . . . . . . . . . . . . . . . . . . . . . . . . . . . . . . . . . . 95
    *Fabrizio Albertetti, Alena Simalastar, and Aïcha Rizzotti-Kaddouri*

Classification of Anxiety Based on EDA and HR . . . . . . . . . . . . . . . . . . 112
    *Raquel Sebastião*

Preliminary Results of IoT-Enabled EDA-Based Analysis of Physiological
Response to Acoustic Stimuli. . . . . . . . . . . . . . . . . . . . . . . . . . . . . . . 124
    *Angelica Poli, Anna Brocanelli, Stefania Cecchi, Simone Orcioni,*
    *and Susanna Spinsante*

## Scenarios and Security

CoviHealth: A Pilot Study with Teenagers in Schools of Centre
of Portugal......................................................... 139
  *María Vanessa Villasana, Ivan Miguel Pires, Juliana Sá,*
  *Nuno M. Garcia, Eftim Zdravevski, Ivan Chorbev, and Petre Lameski*

Dynamic Time Division Scheduling Protocol for Medical Application
Using Frog Synchronization Algorithm ........................... 148
  *Norhafizah Muhammad and Tiong Hoo Lim*

Cybersecurity Analysis for a Remote Drug Dosing and Adherence
Monitoring System ............................................... 162
  *Dino Mustefa and Sasikumar Punnekkat*

**Author Index** .................................................. 179

# Physical Data Tracking Wearables, Applications and Systems

# Development and Evaluation of a Novel Method for Adult Hearing Screening: Towards a Dedicated Smartphone App

Edoardo Maria Polo[1,2], Marco Zanet[3], Marta Lenatti[2], Toon van Waterschoot[4] (ID),
Riccardo Barbieri[2] (ID), and Alessia Paglialonga[3(✉)] (ID)

[1] DIAG, Sapienza University of Rome, 00185 Rome, Italy
[2] Dipartimento di Elettronica, Informazione e Bioingegneria (DEIB), Politecnico di Milano,
20133 Milan, Italy
[3] Institute of Electronics, Information Engineering and Telecommunications (IEIIT),
National Research Council of Italy (CNR), 20133 Milan, Italy
alessia.paglialonga@ieiit.cnr.it
[4] Department of Electrical Engineering (ESAT-STADIUS), KU Leuven, 3001 Leuven, Belgium

**Abstract.** Towards implementation of adult hearing screening tests that can be
delivered via a mobile app, we have recently designed a novel speech-in-noise
test based on the following requirements: user-operated, fast, reliable, accurate,
viable for use by listeners of unknown native language and viable for testing at a
distance. This study addresses specific models to (i) investigate the ability of the
test to identify ears with mild hearing loss using machine learning; and (ii) address
the range of the output levels generated using different transducers. Our results
demonstrate that the test classification performance using decision tree models
is in line with the performance of validated, language-dependent speech-in-noise
tests. We observed, on average, 0.75 accuracy, 0.64 sensitivity and 0.81 specificity.
Regarding the analysis of output levels, we demonstrated substantial variability of
transducers' characteristics and dynamic range, with headphones yielding higher
output levels compared to earphones. These findings confirm the importance of
a self-adjusted volume option. These results also suggest that earphones may not
be suitable for test execution as the output levels may be relatively low, particularly for subjects with hearing loss or for those who skip the volume adjustment
step. Further research is needed to fully address test performance, e.g. testing
a larger sample of subjects, addressing different classification approaches, and
characterizing test reliability in varying conditions using different devices and
transducers.

**Keywords:** Classification · Decision trees · Hearing loss · Hearing screening ·
Smartphone app · Speech-in-noise testing

## 1 Background

The digital health revolution, supported by ubiquitous connectivity, enables new ways
of delivering decentralized healthcare services using eHealth and mHealth solutions,

© ICST Institute for Computer Sciences, Social Informatics and Telecommunications Engineering 2021
Published by Springer Nature Switzerland AG 2021. All Rights Reserved
R. Goleva et al. (Eds.): HealthyIoT 2020, LNICST 360, pp. 3–19, 2021.
https://doi.org/10.1007/978-3-030-69963-5_1

and hearing healthcare makes no exception [1–4]. In the 'new normal' brought by the COVID-19 pandemic, no-touch services are now critical for individuals with age-related hearing loss, who are typically at the highest risk for morbidity and mortality due to their age [5]. In this context, smartphone hearing health apps have grown popular but the availability of validated apps for hearing screening and assessment is still limited [4, 6–8]. Some validated hearing testing apps are currently available on the market, for example *SHOEBOX Audiometry* (an FDA Class II medical device for pure-tone audiometry requiring calibrated transducers) developed by SHOEBOX Ltd, *hearScreen* (a pure-tone audiometry screening app coupled with calibrated headphones), and *hearWHO* (a speech-in-noise testing app, based on the digits-in-noise test [9] in English, endorsed by the World Health Organization), both developed by hearX Group.

Hearing screening in adults is particularly important to identify early signs of hearing loss, and therefore trigger timely intervention, thus preventing or delaying the progression of hearing loss and its impact on communication and psychosocial functioning. In fact, hearing loss is typically neglected in adults and access to care is frequently delayed until major effects in health-related quality of life occur, leading to increased health care costs and utilization patterns [10, 11].

Speech-in-noise tests can be helpful in adult hearing screening to identify the real-life communication problems and to promote awareness in individuals who would otherwise not seek help, or who would seek help very late. Speech-in-noise tests can overcome some of the limitations that make pure-tone audiometry unfeasible for widespread automated self-testing on remote (e.g., need for calibrated transducers, need for low-noise environment) [12, 13]. Moreover, speech-in-noise tests can be easily implemented in an automatic way, for example using multiple-choice tasks on a user-operated interface (e.g., [14–16]). However, a potential limitation of speech-in-noise tests in the context of widespread screening (for example via smartphone apps) is related to the fact that they are typically language-dependent. In fact, these tests typically use sentences, words, or digits and therefore they need to undergo translation, adaptation for psychometric performance, and validation when a new language version has to be developed (e.g., [15, 16]). The use of language-dependent tests may potentially lead to decreased access to screening, disparities, or inaccurate results for non-native listeners and minorities. This is particularly relevant for tests delivered at a distance via smartphone apps as the target population is scattered across native languages.

Recently, we have developed a new and automated speech-in-noise test that reduces possible issues related to language dependence. The test is aimed at adult hearing screening for future implementation in a smartphone app. The main requirements followed for test design are discussed below, along with an outline of the current stage of development:

- *Automated, user-operated execution.* The test is based on a multiple-choice recognition task via an easy-to-use graphical user interface that is optimized for delivery via a touch-sensitive screen. A three-alternative forced-choice task is used with alternatives determined on a maximal opposition criterion (different in place, manner, and voicing) as a proven trade-off between test complexity and psychometric performance [14, 17].
- *Speech stimuli viable for use in individuals of unknown language.* The test is based on meaningless Vowel-Consonant-Vowel (VCV) stimuli spoken by a professional male

native English speaker and a set of consonants common across some of the top spoken languages worldwide (e.g., English, Spanish, French, Portuguese, German, Italian), taking into consideration their viability for application in non-native listeners who are familiar with the Latin alphabet [18, 19]. Preliminary results in native and non-native listeners indicated that the test performance was stable in listeners of varying language [20].

- *Short test duration.* To enable faster convergence of the adaptive algorithm, the test uses a newly developed staircase procedure that, based on the estimated psychometric curves of stimuli, determines optimized upward and downward steps as opposed to conventional staircase procedures that use pre-determined, equal upward and down-ward steps. Preliminary results in normal hearing adults showed that the test duration of the new staircase was, on average, two minutes shorter than that of a conventional staircase (i.e., about 3 min 30 s vs. About 5 min 30 s). Moreover, similar values of test duration were observed in subjects with normal hearing and in subjects with hearing loss [20, 21].

- *Reliable in repeated measures*, to ensure intra-individual repeatability of test results. Preliminary results showed that the proposed test provides repeatable estimates of the speech reception threshold (SRT) and repeatable performance (number of stimuli presented, test duration, and percentage of correct responses) in individuals with normal hearing and with hearing loss. In addition, results showed that, thanks to the short test duration and the multiple-choice design, no perceptual learning effect was observed in the second execution of the test compared to the first one [20, 21].

- *Accurate in identifying hearing loss*, to ensure accurate screening outcomes. Prelim-inary results obtained in a population of 98 adults (including normal hearing and unscreened adults) have shown that, in terms of SRT estimation, the test was as accu-rate as a conventional adaptive staircase [20, 21]. Preliminary analysis of the test classification performance, based on the SRT only, showed that the accuracy (ACC) of the test for the identification of ears with pure-tone thresholds higher than 25 dB HL at 1, 2, or 4 kHz was equal to 0.82 and the area under the receiver operating char-acteristic (AUC) was equal to 0.84 [20]. For a full characterization of classification performance for the purpose of test validation, comprehensive analysis of classifica-tion performance based on the full set of test features (e.g., SRT, number of trials, test duration, percentage of correct responses, average reaction time, and so on) and on a larger sample of individuals is needed. This contribution presents the first results obtained from a multivariate classification approach on a population of 148 adults including subjects with normal hearing and subjects with varying degrees of hearing loss.

- *Viable for testing at a distance*, to ensure reliability of results in varying settings (i.e., in different environments and with different instrumentation). Preliminary results from a group of 26 normal hearing adults showed that the test provided consistent outcomes in terms of SRT estimation and test-retest repeatability in controlled environmental noise settings (audiometer-controlled output levels) and in uncontrolled environmental noise settings (self-adjusted test volume) [21]. However, to fully demonstrate the reliability of test results in varying settings, a deeper analysis of the possible influence of the environmental noise, instrumentation, and test settings is needed. This contribution presents the first results obtained in this direction, specifically a quantitative analysis of the influence of different transducers on the output levels of the test.

Within this context, the aim of this study was twofold. First, regarding the requirement of test accuracy in identifying hearing loss, we performed a preliminary analysis, using a machine learning approach, of the classification performance considering the full set of available features (Sects. 2.2 and 3.1). Second, regarding the requirement of viability for testing at a distance in uncontrolled settings, we conducted an experiment to quantitatively address the influence of self-adjusted test volume settings using different consumer transducers on the output levels of the test (Sects. 2.3 and 3.2). An investigation of these aspects is crucial to fully address the viability of the proposed test for adult hearing screening via a smartphone app.

## 2   Materials and Methods

### 2.1   Speech-in-Noise Test

The proposed speech-in-noise test is based on three-alternative forced-choice recognition of VCV stimuli via a graphical user interface. The set of stimuli includes 12 spoken consonants (/b, d, f, g, k, l, m, n, p, r, s, t/) in the context of the vowel /a/ (e.g., aba, ada) recorded from a male professional native English speaker [14, 20, 21]. VCVs were combined with speech-shaped noise at varying signal-to-noise ratio (SNR). The noise is generated by filtering a Gaussian white noise of amplitude equal to the average level of VCV recordings with the international long-term average speech spectrum [22] and a low-pass filter (cutoff = 1.4 kHz, roll-off slope = 100 dB/octave) and then by adding a noise floor determined by the same filtered noise attenuated by 15 dB [23].

After initial collection of information about the subjects' age and gender through the graphical user interface, the test starts at an initial comfortable level of +8 dB SNR from a stimulus randomly selected from the set of VCVs. Then, it adapts the intelligibility based on a one-up/three-down (1U3D) rule, i.e. the intelligibility is decreased after three correct responses and increased after one incorrect response. The intelligibility is adjusted by changing, concurrently, the VCV and the SNR based on a newly developed staircase procedure [20, 21]. Specifically, the upward and downward steps in SNR are determined adaptively at each trial, based on the psychometric curves of VCV stimuli and therefore the steps depend on the specific stimulus and SNR at each trial. The steps are set using the optimal recommended ratio between downward and upward step size for 1U3D staircases (i.e., 0.74), therefore enabling rapid convergence of the tracking procedure as suggested by [24]. At each step, the VCV presented and the order of the alternatives displayed on the screen are randomized. The procedure is terminated after 12 reversals in SNR and the SRT is estimated as the average of the SNRs at the midpoints of the last four ascending runs [20–24].

### 2.2   Classification Performance

**Participants.** Participants were 148 adults (age = 52.1 ± 20.4 years; age range: 20–89 years; 46 male, 102 female) tested in uncontrolled environmental noise settings in the lab and at local health screening initiatives (i.e. at universities of senior citizens, health prevention and awareness events for the general public). The group of participants included individuals with normal hearing and individuals with varying degrees of hearing impairment. The experimental protocol was approved by the Politecnico di Milano Research Ethical Committee (Opinion n. 2/2019). All subjects were informed about the protocol and the study as a whole and they took part in the experiment on a voluntary basis. Due to the opportunistic nature of the local screening initiatives, participants were given the option to choose in which ear(s) to perform the test. As a result, 8 participants performed the test sequentially in both ears whereas 140 performed the test only in one ear, for a total of 156 ears tested.

**Procedures.** An outline of the experiment is shown in Fig. 1. Participants were tested with: (i) pure-tone audiometry at 0.5, 1, 2, and 4 kHz (Amplaid 177+, Amplifon with TDH49 headphones), and (ii) the proposed speech-in-noise test in uncontrolled environmental noise settings. The test was run on an Apple® Macbook Air® 13″ (OS X Yosemite version 10.10.5 and macOS High Sierra version 10.13.6) connected to Sony MDRZX110APW headphones. The speech-in-noise test was executed in self-adjusted volume settings therefore participants were given the option to adjust the volume at a comfortable level before the test via the graphical user interface.

**Data Analysis.** The pure-tone threshold average (PTA) was computed as the average of hearing thresholds at the four frequencies tested. Then, the tested ears were classified based on their PTA in two classes using the World Health Organization (WHO) criterion for slight/mild hearing impairment: $PTA_{>25 \text{ dB HL}}$ (slight/mild hearing loss) and $PTA_{\leq 25 \text{ dB HL}}$ (no hearing loss) [25]. For a multivariate analysis of the test classification performance, the following features were extracted from the speech-in-noise test software: SRT, total number of trials (#trials), number of correct responses (#correct), percentage of correct responses (%correct), average reaction time (i.e., the average of individual response time throughout the test), test duration, output volume, and age. The eight features extracted from the test were used as input variables of a decision tree (DT) model and the PTA class was used as the output variable (Fig. 1).

A DT approach was used in this first study as it is one of the most broadly used classification methods due to its ability to convert paths in the tree into intelligible decision rules. The Gini index was chosen as splitting rule in place of entropy as they lead to similar results but the Gini index has lower computational weight [26]. To limit the possible effects of overfitting and therefore model bias, the dataset was first split randomly into training (80% of the sample, 124 ears) and test (20% of the sample, 32 ears) datasets. Then, the DT model was optimized using 5-fold cross-validation on the training dataset and finally its predictions were tested on the test dataset. Classification performance was assessed by measuring: accuracy (ACC) on the training and test datasets, area under the curve (AUC), sensitivity (SEN), and specificity (SPE). Due to the relatively small size of the dataset, we also addressed the variability of the model performance. Specifically, we ran 1000 iterations of the model optimization process by randomly changing the initial splitting into training and testing datasets (keeping an 80%/20% splitting ratio) and the inner cross-validation subsets (keeping a 5-fold inner splitting) and then we measured the average and standard deviation of the performance parameters (ACC on the training and test datasets, AUC, SEN, and SPE).

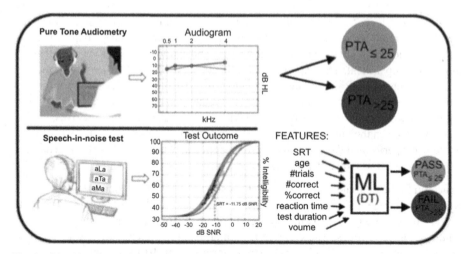

**Fig. 1.** Classification performance analysis methodology. Top panel: Based on the PTA measured with pure-tone audiometry, ears were classified using the WHO criterion for slight/mild hearing impairment as PTA$_{>25\,dB\,HL}$ and PTA$_{\leq25\,dB\,HL}$. Bottom panel: Based on eight features extracted from the speech-in-noise test software, ears were classified into *pass* and *fail* using a DT approach based on the PTA class as the output variable. DT = decision tree; PTA = pure-tone threshold average; WHO = World Health Organization.

### 2.3   Characterization of Transducers

In order to assess the influence of self-adjusted volume settings on the actual output levels of the test, we characterized the performance of different consumer transducers, specifically we measured the actual output levels of the test obtained using a variety of transducers as a function of the self-adjusted test volume settings. In fact, when a screening test is delivered via a smartphone app in uncontrolled environmental noise settings, a variety of transducers can be used therefore it is important to understand the actual output level for a given test volume selected by the user. In this study, we have characterized five different headphones models and two different earphones models widely available on the market, i.e.: Bose Quitecomfort II (in two versions: noise canceling mode ON and noise canceling mode OFF), Sony MDRZX110APW, Sony MDR-7506, Sennheiser PC 310, Akg Y45, Apple EarPods, and Mpow In-ear (price range: 9.99 to 299 €).

The experimental setup for the characterization of transducers is shown in Fig. 2. First, to take into account all the stimuli in the set, an audio file including the sequence of all VCVs, with no pauses, was created. The volume range of the same laptop computer used in the listening tests (described in 1.2) was discretized in 17 levels using a step equal to the size of the volume bars of the laptop. The VCV sequence reproduced via the different transducers, at each of the 17 volume levels, was recorded using a Neumann KU 100 dummy head powered from an external P48 phantom power supply. Each recording was then routed back to the laptop computer via a RME Babyface Pro sound card and the corresponding digital audio files were saved using GarageBand software (version 10.1.3). In order to record the VCV sequence under the same conditions for all the transducers, the dummy head was positioned and remained in the same location in a quiet room and the RME Babyface Pro input gain (dummy head/laptop) was maintained fixed and low throughout the experiment to avoid possible sound saturation.

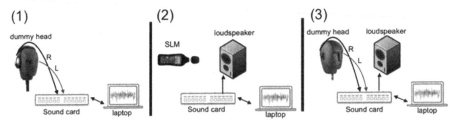

**Fig. 2.** Characterization of transducers. Panel (1): the VCV sequence for each transducer is recorded via a dummy head and a sound card. Panel (2) and (3) show the two steps of the calibration process. Panel (2): the sound card output gain was set to let the white noise from the loudspeaker reach 90 dB SPL on the SLM. Panel (3): the SLM was replaced by the dummy head which recorded the 90 dB SPL white noise and saved it into the laptop maintaining the same input gain of the sound card as that of the VCV sequence recordings. R = right ear; L = left ear; SLM = sound level meter.

A calibration step was needed to convert wave units into dB sound pressure level (SPL). In fact, the absolute amplitude of the recording sequences was in wave units, which are given by the combination of the actual SPL and any other digital gains of the transfer function of the laptop-transducer chain. The calibration process was performed with the dummy head and a loudspeaker and therefore a white noise was used as the recorded loudness of white noise is less influenced by the acoustical attenuation due to the wide frequency range. The white noise was sent via the laptop computer and sound card to the loudspeaker and the loudness was measured using a Sound Level Meter (SLM; Brüel & Kjær Type 2250 Hand Held Analyzer with BZ-7222 Sound Level Meter Software) placed on a tripod in front of the loudspeaker at a distance of 1 m. First, the output gain of the sound card was changed to let the noise loudness reach 90 dB SPL at the SLM. Then, the tripod with the SLM was removed and replaced by the dummy head. Finally, to obtain a calibration factor the white noise was played with the output gain corresponding to a known SLM loudness of 90 dB SPL maintaining the input gain used for the VCV sequence and recorded by the dummy head. The VCV sequences recorded with the different transducers at each of the 17 volume levels were therefore converted in dB SPL and then filtered using an A-weighted filter to approximate the SPL perceived by the average human ear. The experiment was conducted at the Department of Electrical Engineering (ESAT) at KU Leuven.

The characteristics of the transducers, in terms of dB SPL as a function of the volume level were obtained by fitting the 17 sampled measures using polynomial models of order 1–9 using the least-squares method and the optimal model order for each curve was determined using the Akaike information criterion.

# 3 Results

## 3.1 Classification Performance

Figure 3 shows the optimal DT model obtained by using the full set of eight features. Here, it is important to note that, in classifying ears into *pass* or *fail* (as defined by the WHO criterion for slight/mild hearing loss) the top decision node takes into account the value of SRT estimated by the test and uses a cut-off equal to about −7.5 dB SNR to split the tree into branches. On the right-hand side branch, the SRT is also used again down the tree (fourth level split) to classify a subset of 27 ears from subjects older than 58 years (second level split) in which the number of correct responses was lower than or equal to 89 (third level split).

In general, in addition to SRT, the most relevant features for classification are: the subjects' age (with fail outcomes associated with older age), the test duration (totsec in the figure, with fail outcomes associated with longer test duration), and the average reaction time (avg_ans_time in the figure, with fail outcomes associated with longer duration). Splitting rules involving other features such as the total number of correct responses (#correct in the figure), the percentage of correct responses (perc_correct in the figure), or the total number of trials (#trials in the figure) seem to be less informative as rules based on these features are associated with leaf nodes with a very small number of ears (less than 3).

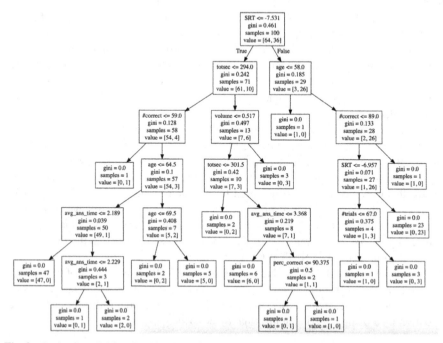

**Fig. 3.** Optimal model for classification of ears into *pass* and *fail* using the full set of features as input variables and the WHO definition of normal hearing/mild hearing loss as output variable.

To address the possible relationships between the model features and their distribution in the two PTA classes, we analyzed the scatter plots for each combination of paired features as well as the distribution of each feature in the two classes. Results are shown in Fig. 4.

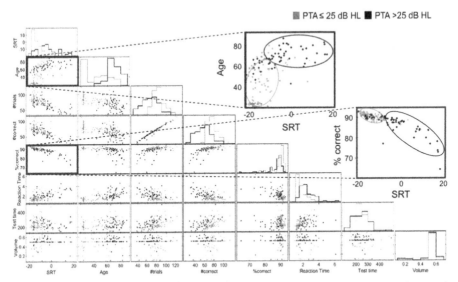

**Fig. 4.** Scatter plots of paired features and, on the diagonal, distributions of single features in the two classes. Magnified versions of two exemplary scatter plots (SRT vs. Age and SRT vs. %correct) are shown on the right-hand side. Green dots: ears with PTA $\leq$ 25 dB HL. Red dots: ears with PTA > 25 dB HL. (Color figure online)

The distributions of each feature, reported on the diagonal of the matrix in Fig. 4, show that some features may be likely candidates for classifying ears in the two PTA classes. Specifically, the better candidates are SRT, age, number of trials and number of correct responses, as well as percentage of correct responses derived from the previous two, and average reaction time. Features such as test duration and volume level show comparable values between the two PTA classes. The scatter plots between pairs of features show that, for example, the SRT combined with features such as age, percentage of correct responses, and average reaction time (as shown in the leftmost column in Fig. 4) generate clusters of data points that are relatively grouped into the two PTA classes, suggesting that a selection of these features may be possibly used to generate simpler DT classification models that are based on a smaller set of rules and may be possibly more intelligible.

To address the performance of models based on a smaller set of rules, we considered DTs with four input features (SRT, age, percentage of correct responses, and average reaction time), as determined by the analysis of the results in Fig. 4. The maximum depth of the DT with four features was set to 4 to counterbalance possible overfitting effects caused by a reduced number of features. The optimal DT model obtained using this selection of features is shown in Fig. 5.

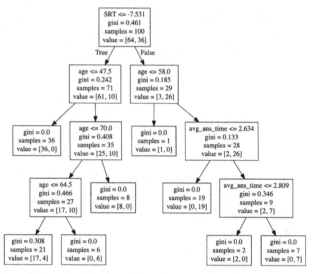

**Fig. 5.** Optimal model for classification of ears into pass and fail using four features as input variables and the WHO definition of normal hearing/mild hearing loss as output variable.

The root node of the DT with four selected features showed in Fig. 5 uses the same rule as the root node of the full model with eight features, i.e. a split on the SRT value using a cut-off equal to −7.5 dB SNR. Noticeably, this cut-off value is close to the cut-off determined in our earlier study using only the SRT on a smaller set of cases, i.e., −8 dB SNR [20]. Importantly, using a generalized linear model with age and SRT as input variables on a dataset of 58 subjects we also showed that, in addition to SRT, the interaction between age and SRT was a significant predictor of PTA class (slight/mild hearing impairment vs no hearing impairment) [27]. This aspect is reflected in the observed DT model as the second most important feature is the subject's age which is used at the second, third, and fourth levels of the tree (Fig. 5). The average reaction time (avg_ans_time in the figure) is also relevant as shown in the right-hand branch of the model at the third and fourth levels of the tree, with fail outcomes associated with lower or alternatively with higher reaction times. In fact, it may be that individuals who have difficulty in speech recognition may just tend to select an alternative on the screen quickly and let the test proceed when they haven't heard the stimulus or, alternatively, it may be that they spend a relatively long time to choose among the alternatives because they are not sure about what they have heard.

Table 1 shows the classification performance and the variability of performance on 1000 iterations (mean ± standard deviation) obtained with the optimal DT models, the one with eight features and the one with four features. The first row shows the accuracy observed in the training dataset ($ACC_{train}$) whereas the remaining rows show the performance (ACC, AUC, SEN, and SPE) observed in the test dataset.

It is important to notice that the two models have slightly different values of ACC on the training and test datasets. For the model with eight features, ACC on the test set is slightly higher than $ACC_{train}$ whereas for the model with four features the opposite

**Table 1.** Classification performance and variability of performance of the optimal DT models with eight input features and with four input features.

| Parameter | Optimal model (8 features) | 1000 iterations (8 features) | Optimal model (4 features) | 1000 iterations (4 features) |
|---|---|---|---|---|
| $ACC_{train}$ | 0.73 | $0.77 \pm 0.0342$ | 0.77 | $0.76 \pm 0.0339$ |
| ACC | 0.78 | $0.76 \pm 0.0721$ | 0.75 | $0.77 \pm 0.0707$ |
| AUC | 0.77 | $0.74 \pm 0.0810$ | 0.72 | $0.75 \pm 0.0803$ |
| SEN | 0.73 | $0.67 \pm 0.1418$ | 0.64 | $0.67 \pm 0.1482$ |
| SPE | 0.81 | $0.81 \pm 0.0895$ | 0.81 | $0.82 \pm 0.0868$ |

trend is observed. However, for each model the mean values of ACC observed on 1000 iterations are similar in the training and testing datasets, and the ACC values are similar between the two models indicating that, overall, the DT classifiers here shown have an average accuracy in the range 0.76 to 0.77, with standard deviation of about 0.07. In general, the observed performance is similar for the DT models with eight and four features in terms of ACC, AUC, SEN, and SPE values. The SEN observed with the optimal model with eight features is seemingly higher than that observed with the optimal model with four features (i.e., 0.73 vs. 0.64). However, the analysis of the mean values obtained on 1000 iterations shows that the average performance of the two models is strikingly similar. Moreover, the observed standard deviations are relatively low for each of the observed performance parameters. The standard deviation is smaller than 0.1 for all the parameters except for sensitivity for which it is about 0.14 and 0.15 for the models with eight and four features, respectively. Therefore, the observed difference in SEN between the two models (0.73 vs. 0.64) may be the result of the inherent variability of the models generated using different distributions of data into the training and test datasets.

### 3.2 Characterization of Transducers

The characteristics of the tested transducers, in terms of dB SPL as a function of volume level (percent value), are shown in Fig. 6. Overall, two different sets of curves were observed for earphones (Apple EarPods and Mpow in-ear) and for headphones. Among the headphones here used, the highest output levels were observed with the Bose Quite-Comfort II headphones with noise canceling mode OFF whereas the characteristics of the remaining headphones were, overall, similar, with differences lower than 6.1 dB SPL across the volume range.

The two tested earphones had an overall linear dynamics and produced lower SPL for a given volume level across the whole volume range. For example, when the volume level is 50% (i.e., the default level on the test software) the output level with the Bose QuiteComfort II headphones with noise canceling mode OFF is about 71.5 dB SPL whereas with Apple ear-pods and Mpow in-ear the output level is about 47.5 and 50 dB SPL, respectively. Similarly, when the volume level is set at the top limit of the range, i.e. at 100% the output level with the Bose QuiteComfort II headphones with noise canceling

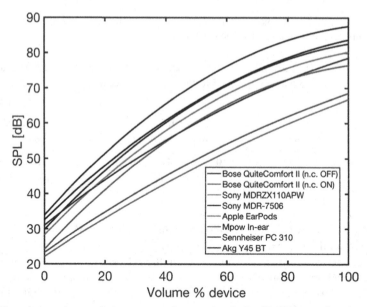

**Fig. 6.** Transducers characteristics: measured output levels (in dB SPL) as a function of laptop volume level (percent value). n.c. = noise canceling.

mode OFF is about 87.5 dB SPL whereas with Apple ear-pods and Mpow in-ear the output level is about 66.5 and 68.5 dB SPL, respectively. The largest differences between transducers were observed at a volume of about 70%, with an observed difference of about 25 dB SPL between Bose QuiteComfort II headphones with noise canceling mode OFF and Apple ear-pods.

## 4   Discussion

In this study, we begun our analysis by addressing classification performance of the proposed speech-in-noise test against the WHO criterion for mild hearing loss using a DT approach in two different configurations: (i) using the full set of eight features (SRT, number of trials, number of correct responses, percentage of correct responses, average reaction time, test duration, output volume, and age) and (ii) using a subset of four features (i.e., SRT, age, percentage of correct responses, and average reaction time) that were selected based on their distributions in the two classes of the output variable.

Overall, the performance of the DT models using eight and four features was similar as shown in Table 1. In addition, the average model performance, determined by running 1000 iterations of model optimization on different realizations of the training and test datasets, was strikingly similar for the DT models with eight and four features in terms of ACC, AUC, SEN, and SPE. The observed variability of performance was also similar between the two models (Table 1).

Compared to the DT model with the full set of eight features, the DT model with four features may have the advantage of being less demanding in terms of computational cost and simpler in terms of interpretability of rules. The DT model with SRT, age, percentage of correct responses, and average reaction time as input features had on the test dataset an ACC equal to 0.75, an AUC equal to 0.72, SEN equal to 0.64 and SPE equal to 0.81. In our earlier analysis of test performance [20], using only the SRT to classify 106 ears from 98 subjects into pass and fail, we observed an ACC equal to 0.82, SEN equal to 0.7, and SPE equal to 0.9 using a cut-off SRT value of -8 dB SNR, i.e. a value close to the cut-off value found in the root nodes of the DT models in this study (Fig. 3, Fig. 5). The AUC measured across the different cut-off SRTs was equal to 0.84 [20]. The values here observed with the DT approach are slightly lower than the values previously observed on a smaller dataset but still in line with the average classification performance of speech-in-noise tests. In general, a moderate level of accuracy is expected due to the inherently different nature of the two hearing tests compared (i.e. pure-tone detection and speech-in-noise recognition), that involve different auditory functions. The performance of other speech-in-noise tests based on multiple-choice recognition of short words is similar or lower than the one here observed. For example, the Earcheck and the Occupational Earcheck (i.e. Internet-based adaptive speech-in-noise tests based on multiple-choice recognition of consonant-vowel-consonant words) had a sensitivity of 0.51 and 0.92 and a specificity of 0.90 and 0.49, respectively, for the detection of ears with noise-induced hearing loss [28]. Similarly, another study on the Occupational Earcheck in a noise-exposed population showed a sensitivity of 0.65 and specificity of 0.63 to detect high-frequency hearing loss above 25 dB HL [29]. Another example is the Speech Understanding in Noise (SUN) test, that uses a list of VCV stimuli in a three-alternatives multiple-choice task presented at predetermined SNRs. The test, when administered sequentially in both ears reached a sensitivity and specificity of about 0.85 for detecting disabling hearing impairment (i.e., PTA > 40 dB HL) [14]. Similarly, the original version of the digits-in-noise test delivered by telephone yielded a sensitivity of 0.75 and a specificity of 0.91 to identify ears with PTA higher than 20.6 dB HL and for the U.S. version of the digits-in-noise test a sensitivity of 0.8 and a specificity of 0.83 to identify ears with PTA higher than 20 dB HL were reported [9, 30]. Therefore, considering the performance of the DT model with four features and the clarity and coherence of the rules generated by this simpler model, so far the DT with SRT, age, percentage of correct responses, and average reaction time as input features is the best candidate model for implementation into the smartphone app for the sake of identifying ears with mild hearing loss.

In the second part of the study, we have analysed the quantitative relationship between the self-adjusted volume levels of the test and the actual output levels in terms of SPL values using a range of consumer transducers, including headphones and earphones. This is relevant for the sake of implementation of a smartphone app as the app may be used with unknown transducers and the actual output levels, i.e. the level at which the speech-in-noise stimuli are delivered to the users' ears, may vary significantly.

Results in Fig. 6 show that the characteristics of different transducers vary greatly across the range of volume levels enabled by the device. The headphones yielded overall higher output SPL compared to earphones, with no substantial differences between types of earphones and types of headphones, except for the Bose QuiteComfort II headphones with noise canceling mode OFF that showed the broadest dynamics and the highest SPL values across the entire volume range of the device.

In general, these results suggest that including the self-adjusted volume option in a future app may help compensate, at least in part, for the different characteristics of the chosen transducer as the subject has the option to set the volume at a comfortable level based on his/her actual loudness perception, which depends on the actual SPL of the stimuli all the other things being equal (hearing sensitivity, mobile device characteristics, transducer, and environmental noise levels). This provides further support to the choice of including a self-adjusted volume option to enable test delivery via a mobile app in uncontrolled environment and with unknown transducers.

The results in Fig. 6 also point out that the range of output SPLs that can be generated with earphones is, in general, narrower than the one that can be obtained with headphones, with earphones providing much lower SPL values than headphones – up to about 20–25 dB SPL lower when a volume in the range 50–70% is used. This means that, even by using the full range of available output levels, the maximum SPL that can be obtained by using the tested earphones will be between 65 and 70 dB. As a benchmark, conversational speech occurs at an average of 65 dB SPL with a typical dynamic range of 30 dB (12 dB above and 18 dB below the average) [31, 32]. Therefore, the maximum SPL reached by the earphones models here tested might not be sufficient to provide clearly intelligible speech stimuli to subjects with reduced hearing sensitivity due hearing loss. For example, subjects with minimal hearing loss as defined by the WHO criterion would hear the test sounds attenuated by an average of 25 dB and the perceived sounds will be even weaker in case of mild or moderate hearing losses with higher PTA. For example, in case of PTA equal to 25 dB HL (which is the lowest PTA in the mild hearing loss range), a sound at 70 dB SPL would be perceived, on average, in a similar way as a sound of 45 dB SPL, a level that corresponds to faint speech and that would be therefore barely perceivable. Moreover, it may also happen that some of the tested subjects may not wish to adjust the device volume, as we observed for example in our listening tests. In fact, the average volume measured in our experiments was 0.48 (standard deviation = 0.11) and 83 out of 48 participants left the volume unchanged to the default value of 50%. Therefore, these results indicate that it may be important to recommend that headphones are used rather than earphones in combination with the smartphone testing app.

## 5  Limitations and Future Work

This study provided promising results but it has some limitations. First, the values of performance observed following a single model optimization process are slightly different than the average performance estimated across several iterations of the process, as shown in Table 1. This discrepancy is mainly due to the limited size of our dataset therefore it happens that a single optimized model may not accurately reflect the potential performance of the method in this task. Future studies will be necessary, on a significantly larger sample of adults and older adults, to increase the sample size and therefore improve the quality of the classifier developed before the algorithm can be safely implemented into a mobile app.

Second, in this study we investigated only one type of classification algorithm, the DT, due to its widespread use and its ability to generate intelligible decision rules. However, to fully explore the potential of multivariate classification algorithms for the identification of hearing loss and the possible advantages of machine learning methods over univariate classification approaches further research is needed. For example, it will be important to test different DT models by varying the set of input features and different machine learning algorithms, including both explainable (rule-based) and black-box approaches. The final outcome of this future investigation will be the identification of an optimal classification model that is accurate and reliable in identifying ears with hearing loss and that can be implemented into a smartphone app as part of the testing software.

In addition, the test partially addresses the problem of language-dependence. On the one hand, the use of meaningless VCVs and a set of consonants that is common across some of the top spoken languages worldwide makes the test feasible for use in non-native listeners. On the other hand, listeners who are not familiar with the Latin alphabet or native listeners of character-based languages such as Mandarin or Japanese may be subjected to ambiguities arising from the phoneme-grapheme correspondence. Investigation of test performance in a larger sample of native languages would be important to understand the possible modifications needed to improve test validity on a broader population.

Although we are getting very close to our final goal, further research is still needed to fully define the optimal settings for test delivery via a smartphone app. For example, it will be important to measure the output levels obtained using mobile devices to understand the potential output levels range that can be obtained using a smartphone or a tablet device. Moreover, it will be useful to address the characteristics of additional transducers, including additional earphones models with broader dynamic range, to understand which models are more suited for test execution and define minimum requirements for transducers to be used in the test in uncontrolled environmental conditions.

## 6   Conclusions

In this study, we have shown that an approach based on explainable machine learning using a decision tree algorithm in combination with the proposed speech-in-noise test can classify ears with similar accuracy, sensitivity, and specificity as that of popular validated speech-in-noise tests. Moreover, we have shown that a simplified classification model with a reduced set of features can lead to simpler, more intelligible rules and maintain the same performance of more complex models based on a larger set of input features. Regarding the analysis of the output levels of the test as a function of different transducers, we have highlighted important differences in output levels between types of transducers (headphones vs. earphones) as well as between different transducer models, also showing that some transducers may not be adequate to ensure an appropriate range of output levels for the sake of conducting the test in self-adjusted volume settings. Further research will be needed to fully address the accuracy of the test, specifically it will be important to collect data from a larger sample of subjects, to evaluate the performance of different machine learning algorithms, preferably those able to generate explainable (e.g., rule-based) models, and to characterize the reliability of the test in varying environmental noise conditions and using different devices.

**Acknowledgement.** The research leading to these results has received funding from the European Research Council under the European Union's Horizon 2020 research and innovation program or

ERC Consolidator Grant: SONORA (773268). This article reflects only the authors' views, and the Union is not liable for any use that may be made of the contained information.

The authors are grateful to the Lions Clubs International and to Associazione La Rotonda, Baranzate (MI) for their support in the organization and management of experiments in the unscreened population of adults. The authors wish to thank Anna Bersani, Carola Butera, and Antonio Carrella from Politecnico di Milano who helped with data collection at Associazione La Rotonda. The Authors would also like to thank Dr. Randall Ali from the Department of Electrical Engineering at KU Leuven for providing guidance during the transducers characterization experiment.

# References

1. Swanepoel, D.W.: eHealth technologies enable more accessible hearing care. In: Seminars in Hearing, vol. 41, no. 02, pp. 133–140 (2020)
2. Paglialonga, A.: eHealth and mHealth for audiologic rehabilitation. In: Montano, J.J., Spitzer, J.B. (eds.) Adult Audiologic Rehabilitation, 3rd edn. Plural Publishing, San Diego (2020)
3. Paglialonga, A., Cleveland Nielsen, A., Ingo, E., Barr, C., Laplante-Lévesque, A.: eHealth and the hearing aid adult patient journey: a state-of-the-art review. BioMed. Eng. Online 17, 101 (2018)
4. Paglialonga, A., Tognola, G., Pinciroli, F.: Apps for hearing science and care. Am. J. Audiol. 24(3), 293–298 (2015)
5. Audiology Today: Tele-audiology in a Pandemic and Beyond: Flexibility and Suitability in Audiology Practice. https://www.audiology.org/audiology-today-julyaugust-2020/tele-aud iology-pandemic-and-beyond-flexibility-and-suitability. Accessed 24 July 2020
6. Bright, T., Pallawela, D.: Validated smartphone-based apps for ear and hearing assessments: a review. JMIR Rehabil. Assist. Tech. 3(2), e13 (2016)
7. Colsman, A., Supp, G.G., Neumann, J., Schneider, T.R.: Evaluation of accuracy and reliability of a mobile screening audiometer in normal hearing adults. Front. Psychol. 11, 744 (2020)
8. De Sousa, K.C., Swanepoel, D.W., Moore, D.R., Smits, C.: A smartphone national hearing test: performance and characteristics of users. Am. J. Audiol. 27(3S), 448–454 (2018)
9. Smits, A., Kapteyn, T., Houtgast, T.: Development and validation of an automatic speech-in-noise screening test by telephone. Int. J. Audiol. 43, 1–28 (2004)
10. Nachtegaal, J., Festen, J.M., Kramer, S.E.: Hearing ability and its relationship with psychosocial health, work-related variables, and health care use: the national longitudinal study on hearing. Audiol. Res. 1(1), e9 (2011)
11. Reed, N.S., et al.: Trends in health care costs and utilization associated with untreated hearing loss over 10 years. JAMA Otolaryngol. Head Neck Surg. 145(1), 27–34 (2019)
12. Humes, L.E.: Understanding the speech-understanding problems of older adults. Am. J. Audiol. 22(2), 303–305 (2013)
13. Killion, M.C., Niquette, P.A., Gudmundsen, G.I., Revit, L.J., Banerjee, S.: Development of a quick speech-in-noise test for measuring signal-to-noise ratio loss in normal-hearing and hearing-impaired listeners. J. Acoust. Soc. Am. 116, 2395–2405 (2004)
14. Paglialonga, A., Tognola, G., Grandori, F.: A user-operated test of suprathreshold acuity in noise for adult hearing screening: the SUN (Speech Understanding in Noise) test. Comput. Biol. Med. 52, 66–72 (2014)
15. Jansen, S., Luts, H., Wagener, K.C., Frachet, B., Wouters, J.: The French digit triplet test: a hearing screening tool for speech intelligibility in noise. Int. J. Audiol. 49(5), 378–387 (2010)

16. Potgieter, J.M., Swanepoel, W., Myburgh, H.C., Smits, C.: The South African English smart-phone digits-in-noise hearing test: effect of age, hearing loss, and speaking competence. Ear Hear. **39**(4), 656–663 (2019)
17. Leek, M.R.: Adaptive procedures in psychophysical research. Percept. Psychophys. **63**(8), 1279–1292 (2001)
18. Cooke, M., Lecumberri, M.L.G., Scharenborg, O., van Dommelen, W.A.: Language-independent processing in speech perception: identification of English intervocalic consonants by speakers of eight European languages. Speech Commun. **52**, 954–967 (2010)
19. Rocco G.: Design, implementation, and pilot testing of a language-independent speech intelligibility test. M.Sc. thesis dissertation, Department of Electronics Information and Bioengineering, Politecnico di Milano, Milan, Italy (2018)
20. Paglialonga, A., Polo, E.M., Zanet, M., Rocco, G., van Waterschoot, T., Barbieri, R.: An automated speech-in-noise test for remote testing: development and preliminary evaluation. Am. J. Audiol. **29**(3S), 564–576 (2020)
21. Zanet, M., Polo, E.M., Rocco, G., Paglialonga, A., Barbieri, R.: Development and preliminary evaluation of a novel adaptive staircase procedure for automated speech-in-noise testing. In: Proceedings of the 41st Annual International Conference of the IEEE Engineering in Medicine and Biology Society (EMBC) (2019)
22. Byrne, D., et al.: An international comparison of long-term average speech spectra. J. Acoust. Soc. Am. **96**(4), 2108–2120 (1994)
23. Leensen, M.C., de Laat, J.A., Snik, A.F., Dreschler, W.A.: Speech-in-noise screening tests by Internet, part 2: improving test sensitivity for noise-induced hearing loss. Int. J. Audiol. **50**(11), 835–848 (2011)
24. García-Pérez, M.A.: Forced-choice staircases with fixed step sizes: asymptotic and small-sample properties. Vision. Res. **38**(12), 1861–1881 (1998)
25. World Health Organization (WHO): Grades of hearing impairment. https://www.who.int/pbd/deafness/hearing_impairment_grades/en/#. Accessed 02 Aug 2020
26. Raileanu, L.E., Stoffel, K.: Theoretical comparison between the Gini index and information gain criteria. Ann. Math. Artif. Intell. **41**, 77–93 (2004)
27. Polo, E.M., Zanet, M., Paglialonga, A., Barbieri, R.: Preliminary evaluation of a novel language independent speech-in-noise test for adult hearing screening. In: Jarm, T., Cvetkoska, A., Mahnič-Kalamiza, S., Miklavcic, D. (eds.) EMBEC 2020. IP, vol. 80, pp. 976–983. Springer, Cham (2021). https://doi.org/10.1007/978-3-030-64610-3_109
28. Leensen, M.C., de Laat, J.A., Dreschler, W.A.: Speech-in-noise screening tests by Internet, part 1: test evaluation for noise-induced hearing loss identification. Int. J. Audiol. **50**(11), 823–834 (2011)
29. Sheikh Rashid, M., Dreschler, W.A.: Accuracy of an Internet-based speech-in-noise hearing screening test for high-frequency hearing loss: incorporating automatic conditional rescreening. Int. Arch. Occup. Environ. Health **91**(7), 877–885 (2018)
30. Watson, C., Kidd, G., Miller, J., Smits, C., Humes, L.: Telephone screening tests for functionally impaired hearing: current use in seven countries and development of a US version. J. Am. Acad. Audiol. **23**(10), 757–767 (2012)
31. Accredited Standards Committee S3, Bioacoustics. ANSI S3.5–1997. Methods for Calculation of the Speech Intelligibility Index. American National Standards Institute, New York (1997)
32. Pearsons, K.S., Bennett, R.L., Fidell, S.: Speech Levels in Various Noise Environments. US Environmental Agency, Office of Health and Ecological Effects, Office of Research and Development, Washington, DC (1977).

# A Non-invasive Cloud-Based IoT System and Data Analytics Support for Women Struggling with Drug Addictions During Pregnancy

Victor Balogun[1]([✉]), Oluwafemi A. Sarumi[2], and Oludolapo D. Balogun[3]

[1] Department of Applied Computer Science, University of Winnipeg,
Winnipeg, Canada
vi.balogun@uwinnipeg.ca
[2] Department of Computer Science, The Federal University of Technology,
Akure, Nigeria
oasarumi@futa.edu.ng
[3] Department of Community Health Sciences, University of Manitoba,
Winnipeg, Canada
balogu12@myumanitoba.ca

**Abstract.** Drug abuse among pregnant women and the subsequent neonatal illness are very crucial clinical and social problems. Drugs misuse during pregnancy places the mother and her baby at increased risk of severe complications including deformities, low birth weight, and mental disabilities. Pregnancy can motivate a woman to enter into an addiction treatment program to protect her unborn baby from the effects of drug misuse. Despite the availability of several treatment centers, many women do not seek needed help during and after pregnancy. Some of the reasons include stigmatization, fear of their babies being taken away by Child and Family Services, and the fear of confinement to a facility. In this paper, we propose a non-invasive Cloud-based Internet-of-Things (IoT) and Data Analytics framework that will provide support for women seeking addiction treatment during pregnancy. The system will use simplified sensors incorporated into a smartwatch to monitor, collect, and process vital data from pregnant women to identify instances of emergencies. During emergencies, the system automatically contacts specific needed service(s) and sends the processed data to the cloud for storage and Data Analytics to provide deeper insight and necessary decision making. The framework ensures that pregnant women are not confined into a facility and are reachable remotely by healthcare practitioners during addiction treatment. These capabilities guarantee that the system is operational during global pandemics like COVID-19. The framework integrates every patient's data into a centralized database accessible to all healthcare practitioners thereby preventing multiple prescriptions of the same medication by different doctors.

**Keywords:** Drug addiction · Pregnant women · IoT · Cloud · Fog · Healthcare · WBAN

© ICST Institute for Computer Sciences, Social Informatics and Telecommunications Engineering 2021
Published by Springer Nature Switzerland AG 2021. All Rights Reserved
R. Goleva et al. (Eds.): HealthyIoT 2020, LNICST 360, pp. 20–34, 2021.
https://doi.org/10.1007/978-3-030-69963-5_2

# 1   Introduction

The unprecedented increase in drug abuse among pregnant women in recent time and the ensuing neonatal illness are very crucial clinical and social concerns. Any pregnant woman that wants to give birth to a healthy baby devoid of medical problems must ensure that she promotes a healthy pregnancy. The possibility of having a healthy baby is drastically reduced if such a woman uses illegal drugs and does not seek addiction treatment during pregnancy. The use of drugs during pregnancy can lead to fetal growth limitations such as diminished body mass and other medical difficulties including preterm birth and infectious diseases. Poole [11] reported that when the fetus is exposed to alcohol, it can lead to varieties of undesirable consequences collectively known as fetal alcohol spectrum disorder, including fetal alcohol syndrome (FAS). The same report stated that FAS occurs at a rate of one to two cases per 1,000 live births in Canada. Some of the manifestations of FAS in births include facial abnormalities, growth deficiencies and damage to the central nervous system. When pregnant women use cocaine, it can lead to narrowing of blood vessels in the uterus and placenta, with the eventual result of malnourished fetal growth [5]. Children given birth to by mothers having issues with addictions suffer from postnatal issues including poor parenting, neglect, abuse, mental illness, and in some cases death. Therefore, there is a need to effectively address these complex prenatal and postnatal problems so as to provide help needed by pregnant women struggling with addictions and their unborn babies.

The importance of addiction treatments for women struggling with drug misuse during pregnancy cannot be overemphasized. Finnegan *et al.* [5], observed that when pregnant women struggling with drug addictions are supported with treatments, they are more likely to give birth to children with lesser birth defects. Over the years, several addiction centers have been set up by both private and public initiatives so as to support individuals struggling with different categories of substance misuse. Pregnancy period has been deemed as a time of increased motivation for women to enter into an addiction treatment program so as to protect their unborn babies from the effects of drug misuse. Despite the availability of these treatment centers, many of these women do not seek needed help during and after pregnancy. Some of the reasons given by such women include stigmatization as a result of their addictive behaviors, fear of their babies being taken away by Child and Family Services (CFS), the fear of being confined to a facility during addiction treatments, lack of access to specific treatment programs for addiction during pregnancy, and lack of support from partners or family members. Finnegan [3] reiterated that the fear of stigmatization makes women reluctant in seeking help with their addictions and when they do, they meet with obstacles that make it difficult for them to obtain needed medical and obstetrical services. Such obstacles include misinformation, denials, and unresponsiveness of the health service providers. In recent time, with the onset of the COVID-19 pandemic, continuous access of pregnant women seeking addiction treatment to healthcare services has been greatly impacted. The concepts of social distancing and working from home have further contributed to lack of access to such services.

## 2   Problem Statement - Pregnant Women and Drug Addiction

Close to 3% of the 4.1 million women in the United States that are within the childbearing age but abuse drugs are believed to keep on using drugs even when pregnant [8]. The United States' 2010 National Survey on Drug Use and Health (NSDUH) stated that 4.4% of pregnant women between the age of 15–44 years reported illicit drug use [12]. According to the 2006–2007 Maternity Experience Survey done in Canada, 10.5% of women smoked cigarettes daily or occasionally during the last three months of pregnancy, 10.5% drank alcohol during their pregnancy, and 1% used street drugs while pregnant [11]. In [10], Reproductive Health Working Group in Alberta reported that 2.3% of women who gave birth to live infants in 2006 used illicit drugs during pregnancy. On the national level, [16] stated that the 2008 Canadian Perinatal Health Report shows that 11% of pregnant women consumed alcohol while 5% of women used illegal drugs during pregnancy. Another report by [7] revealed that in the previous year, among Canadian women of childbearing age, 76.7% consumed alcohol, about 11% used cannabis, and 2.1% used illicit drugs including cocaine, ecstasy, speed, hallucinogens and heroin during pregnancy.

The effect of drug misuse during pregnancy both on the mother and the unborn baby cannot be overemphasized. Center for Behavioral Health Statistics and Quality [26] reported that about 7 million people in 2015 suffer from illegal drug use disorder while about one to four deaths were attributed to drug misuse, tobacco and alcohol. But it was estimated by the same report that only about 14% of adults with illegal drug use disorder actually received treatments within the year. The author in [3] stated that when pregnant women engage in drug misuse, it places the mother at increased risk of several childbirth complications including early pregnancy loss, premature detachment of the placenta from the wall of the uterus, placental insufficiency, sudden rise in blood pressure, convulsions or coma, premature labor, premature rupture of membranes, and postpartum hemorrhage. Apart from the effect of drug addiction on the mother and child, Florence et al. [27] stated that misuse of prescription opioid costs the U.S. economy more than 78.5 billion every year.

### 2.1   Notable Signs of Drug Misuse in Pregnant Women

Pregnant women and other people struggling with illicit drug addictions irrespective of the type of the drug can be distinguished using some pathological set of behaviors that associate with the misuse of any illegal drug. American Addiction Centers [24], grouped these behaviors into four main categories including impaired control, social impairment, risky use and pharmacological indicators (tolerance and withdrawal). **Impaired control** of substance includes evidence of someone using a larger amount of a substance than intended, using it for an extended period than intended, and uncontrolled cravings for the substance such that the user is unable to function or think of anything else. **Social impairment** is characterized by sets of harmful behaviors exhibited as a result of repeated use of a substance. Evidence of this includes people continuously using substances even when the usage has caused them their jobs, families, friendships and other social responsibilities. Such a one might also give up or reduce important recreational activities like playing sports with friends. **Risky use** of substances is manifested when substance users continued with the usage of drugs despite the harm they experienced. Such a one continued to use the substance despite they are in physically hazardous scenarios like driving a car, continuous smoking of cigarettes even though the abuser is experiencing respiratory problems and continuous drinking of alcohol even when a pregnant woman knows that it is dangerous for the fetus. The last notable sign of drug misuse in people including pregnant women is categorized as **pharmacological indicators**. This has to do with the level of adjustment that the body makes so as to tolerate frequent misuse of drugs. When someone has developed tolerance for a drug, the body will respond to a drastic stoppage of the drug by exhibiting withdrawal symptoms. These symptoms could be very fatal and as such, pregnant women attempting to stop the misuse of illicit drugs need medical support and other related support systems so as not to endanger the health of the fetus.

As reported by [24], for example, withdrawal from cocaine misuse is normally demonstrated in three major phases including initial crash, acute withdrawal and extinction period. The initial crash period is characterized by extended sleeping, increase in appetite and the feeling of depression or agitation of the individual with the cocaine addiction. The acute withdrawal period is characterized by periods of sleeplessness, anxiety, fatigue and irritability. While the extinction period climaxed with the thought of suicide and intense cravings for cocaine which might continue for several months even after the stoppage of cocaine. As further explained in the same report, withdrawal from alcohol has varieties of side effects including seizures, fever, severe confusion, hallucinations, agitation, fatigue, muscle aches, loss of appetite, dizziness and sleeplessness to mention a few. Finnegan *et al.* [4] reported that medical issues perceived in babies delivered by heroin-addicted mothers are functions of the quantity of prenatal care received by the mother as well as the level of exposure of the fetus to drugs from the mother during pregnancy. The authors stated that when a pregnant woman is exposed to multiple drugs, it can lead to overdose and complicated withdrawal symptoms that can endanger the health of the woman as well as the fetus. Therefore, it is important that pregnant women exhibiting these symptoms are provided with immediate medical attention and other necessary support to prevent further fatalities.

## 2.2 Classifying Addictions in Pregnant Women and Identifying Level of Prenatal and Postnatal Support Needed

Addictions in pregnant women or in any other people can be classified into three different levels based on the ability to carry on with day-to-day activities. These include functional, semi-functional and non-functional addictions. We use this simplified taxonomy with the intent of describing the functional level of the addicted pregnant women with respect to their ability to go about their daily activities. This will help us to determine the level of support needed as they undergo addiction treatment during and after pregnancy. These classifications closely agree with the taxonomy presented in [15] where substance use disorder was described using three sub-classifications including mild addiction, moderate addiction and severe addiction.

The pregnant women that fall within the category of **functional** (mild) addiction are those that though they use illicit drugs and may sometimes experience overdose, but they are able to carry on with their day-to-day activities including maintaining a job or profession, maintaining a shelter, attending medical related appointments and are able to control their behaviors during drug misuse. At the other end of the addiction spectrum is the **non-functional** (severe) addicted pregnant woman. These women lose total control of themselves when using illicit drugs and as such they are not able to maintain a job, accommodation or provide the basic necessity of life to keep themselves and their unborn babies healthy during and after pregnancy. These categories of women are the most vulnerable as they have the tendency to exhibit all the negative effects of drug addiction both in the pregnant mother and their babies. They are mostly homeless, malnourished and needing intensive medical attention during and after pregnancy. At the center of the addiction spectrum is yet another level of addiction which we refer to as **semi-functional** (moderate) addiction. The women in this class of addiction are able to carry out some basic activities of life but with close supervision or support from other people. These women might be in and out of jobs frequently as a result of their addictive tendencies, they could also be homeless most times or needing help to live with friends and family members. They cannot be relied on to keep medical appointments or to maintain a daily schedule that will be advantageous to their health and that of their unborn babies.

## 2.3 Supporting Addicted Pregnant Women - Issues and Challenges

Misuse of illegal drugs in pregnant women can be very challenging to treat by the current healthcare system. The fact that there are different levels of drug addictions in pregnant women suggests that they will require different levels of support system. Therefore, there is a need to develop a holistic treatment approach and integrated support services that consider the level of support needed by the addicted mother during treatment without adverse effect on both mother and child. Finnegan [3] confirmed that the pregnancy is a period of increased motivation for women to enter into an addiction treatment program. Despite this, many pregnant women do not enter into addiction recovery programs during pregnancy.

Some of the reasons emanate from the discrimination and stigmatization experienced by pregnant women as a result of their addictive behaviors. This can create a huge barrier to engaging in prenatal care and drug misuse treatment programs. Some other reasons why pregnant women do not seek addiction treatment during pregnancy include illiteracy, fear of their babies being taken away by Child and Family Services (CFS), the fear of being confined to a facility during addiction treatments, lack of information about and access to specific treatment programs for addiction during pregnancy, and lack of support from their partners or family members.

# 3  Method of Solution - IoT Support for Drug Addicted Pregnant Women

The goal of this research is to use a lightweight IoT (Internet of Things)-based wearable device (smartwatch) to support pregnant women struggling with drug addiction with the intent of providing them with access to real-time medical support especially during emergencies and global pandemics like COVID-19. The wearable device, with the aid of the inbuilt sensors will be used to monitor and collect vital data such as blood pressure, heartbeat rate, movement pattern, and body temperature from the pregnant women. The data collected could be immediately processed using the mobile phone of the pregnant woman or could be processed using an edge/fog computing device. The basic data analytics can be performed at this level to determine if the user is in need of urgent medical assistance. When there is an emergency, the mobile phone or edge device will alert the necessary emergency service(s) automatically so as to immediately attend to the need of the pregnant woman. The major advantage of this approach is that the technology will allow pregnant women struggling with addiction to go through a rehabilitation process without being confined to a controlled facility. In addition, location data collected through the sensors embedded into the smartwatch of a pregnant woman can be used to enhance an automated contact tracing system for anyone that has been in close contact with any pregnant women showing symptoms of COVID-19. In the rest of this paper, we will present the details of the different technologies and techniques of our proposed approach, the challenges of using this approach to support pregnant women struggling with addictions and how to overcome these challenges.

## 3.1  IoT in Health-Care

Fan *et al.* [20] described the Internet of Things (IoT) as a network consisting of several devices interacting together in a machine to machine communications with the aim of collection and exchange of data. IoT and the development of other wireless technologies like Wireless Body Area Network (WBAN), have been earmarked as potential solutions for enabling patient's health monitoring applications that can be streamlined in real-time to health practitioners, especially during emergency [19]. WBAN is the intercommunication of several wearable or implanted mobile sensors with the aim of collecting vital data from the body to a home base station where it can be processed and sent to a health center for needed care [16]. Certain human body parameters including movement pattern, heart rate, blood pressure, body temperature and respiration rate can be measured by sensors and portable devices without human intervention [14].

With the increasing support and integration of IoT in healthcare services and applications, handling the massive healthcare data that need to be stored, secured, managed and exchanged between devices, and accessed ubiquitously can be very challenging. A potential solution to overcoming these challenges is the use of Cloud computing. Cloud computing in recent times has become a de facto standard for providing on-demand computing resources because of its mobility, scalability and security. Cloud computing can be used as a backbone network to provide storage and network services to support IoT healthcare systems [22]. Recently, there is an increasing change in computing paradigm from centralized (Cloud) computing to decentralized (Fog/Edge) computing [23]. The concept of Fog or Edge computing was first introduced by CISCO as they attempt to provide a network solution that extends the computing power and storage capability of the Cloud closer to the edge of the WBAN [21]. Fog computing brings the Cloud closer to the network users, thereby enabling the collection, storage and local processing of data. The advantages of Fog computing include real-time processing, reduced network latency, improved data privacy and reduced cost of implementation [14].

## 3.2  Related Work

In this section, we present a review of some research that has been done that has close connection with our proposed system. The intent of this review is to analyze what has been done with respect to IoT for healthcare delivery, so as to identify why the current systems are not suitable to provide technological-based support for pregnant women struggling with drug addiction. Baker *et al.* [1], described generally the basic elements of an IoT in the healthcare system. The authors introduce a framework that can be used in various IoT for healthcare applications without particular reference to how to apply it in supporting pregnant women with drug addiction. Farahani *et al.* [2], introduced a systematic IoT e-health ecosystem made up of hardware and software devices without a specific implementation of such IoT models. Kumari *et al.* [9] presented a three-layer healthcare architecture for real-time applications that includes a fog computing layer. The authors further addressed the opportunities and challenges of implementing such IoT-enabled architecture for health service delivery. In [13], the authors presented an IoT system that can collect data about patient health status through multiple sensors and the data collected can be conveyed to a remote server for real-time analysis. [6] proposed a fog computing-based framework which was applied on a prototype so as to accelerate the response to mobile patients.

Dang *et al.* [14] described a system where a network of connected sensors record a patient's vitals and the data is continuously sent to a broker. The broker in turn analyzes and stores processed data on the cloud. The system allows a subscriber to directly monitor patients from any location and to respond immediately to emergencies. The system was not investigated for supporting sensitive applications like the monitoring of pregnant women with addiction problems in which the patients cannot be attached with sensors that can easily be detached from the body during a medical crisis. There is a need to investigate a framework that uses sensors that are embedded within mobile devices that are normally worn by users (e.g. smartwatch) and not an extra attachment or carry on for the user. Pasluosta *et al.* [17] investigated an IoT technology for monitoring patients suffering from Parkinson's Disease. The author concluded that wearable sensors for observing gait patterns, tremors, and general activity levels could be used in combination with vision-based technologies (i.e. cameras) around the home to monitor progression of Parkinson's Disease. This work only investigated IoT for Parkinson's Disease and there is no significant correlation with application that involved monitoring addiction in pregnant women. In [25], an ECG sensor was used to measure heart activity of patients using a microcontroller. Though the authors suggested that such a system could be used to predict incidents of heart attack, the bulkiness of the system makes it unsuitable for use in monitoring addicted pregnant women.

## 4   Cloud-Based IoT Support for Drug Addicted Pregnant Women

Healthcare support and monitoring system that confines the user to a restricted facility is not desirable for supporting the different categories of addicted pregnant women requiring different levels of support. The functional addicted women are able to go about their daily activities despite their momentary addiction tendencies and as such should not be confined to a facility for addiction treatment. In addition, IoT systems that use sensors implemented on a circuit board that needs to be attached to the body or sensors that need to be attached to different parts of the body are also not desirable for supporting addicted pregnant women. This is because, the sensors will constitute as extra weight or object that the pregnant women might find inconvenient to carry around. When a pregnant woman is also going through a crisis due to addiction, the attached sensors could be easily stripped off by the pregnant women, leading to monitoring failure.

In order to solve the problems associated with monitoring addicted pregnant women, we propose an IoT-enabled healthcare support system that uses a smartwatch that is normally worn by the user. The smartwatch is embedded with essential sensors that are needed to monitor the behavior of the pregnant woman during drug overdose or when exhibiting withdrawal symptoms. This approach will provide the pregnant women with a non-intrusive and portable monitoring system that allows the users to go about their day-to-day activities while receiving addiction treatment. Another advantage is that the pregnant women will find addiction treatment services more accessible and attractive since they are not confined to a place or required to carry around a heavy monitoring device. Likewise, the approach disallows the embedding of monitoring sensors under the skin of pregnant women. To the best of our knowledge, this will be the first time that a non-invasive Cloud-based IoT healthcare service delivery is being considered for supporting pregnant women struggling with drug misuse.

The architecture of our proposed IoT-enabled healthcare system is presented in Fig. 1. The body sensors embedded within the smartwatch constantly monitor and collect pregnant women health parameters including movement pattern, body temperature, blood pressure and heart rate. The data collected are sent to the user's mobile phone where it is temporarily stored and analyzed before it is sent to the cloud for permanent storage and further processing. If a health concern or emergency incident is detected when the data is processed within the mobile phone, the mobile phone will automatically alert the respective health service provider needed to support the pregnant woman at that instance. Alternatively, instead of using the mobile phone for processing, the collected data can be sent by the mobile phone to an edge or fog computing device where it can be analyzed to provide real-time support for the user. As a result of this design, the health caregivers are able to monitor pregnant women remotely and are able to respond in a timely manner to crisis and emergencies due to drug misuse.

## 5    The Architecture of IoT Support for Drug Addicted Pregnant Women

The architecture presented in Fig. 1 is a four-layer architecture consisting of the sensor/WBAN layer, the personal server/fog computing layer, the cloud computing layer and the medical service layer.

### 5.1    Sensor or WBAN Layer

The Sensor or WBAN layer is where health-related data are collected from the body of the users with the aid of sensors embedded within the smartwatch worn by the users. [1,18] identify some portable sensors that can be used for collecting data from users in a WBAN. Some of the sensors that we consider relevant to collecting data related to drug addiction behavior in pregnant women include the Accelerometer for measuring body movement so as to track users steps and sleeping patterns, Heart Rate monitor, EMG (electromyography) sensor for monitoring muscle activity, Oximetry sensor for measuring blood oxygen which is the key to reporting accurate pulse rates, skin conductance sensor for measuring the galvanic skin response or how much a user sweats, Blood Pressure sensor, skin temperature sensor for monitoring user's body temperature and GPS to identify user's current location.

## 5.2    Personal Server/Fog Computing Layer

The Personal Server or Fog Computing layer is the link between the Sensor layer, the Medical Service layer and the Cloud Computing layer. The health-related data collected by the sensors are sent using the short-range Zigbee or Bluetooth wireless technologies to the pregnant women smartphone which will serve as the gateway. An example of such a gateway is the Android gateway [34] which enables local storage and pre-processing of data collected from the WBAN sensors. This layer can be implemented using a cell phone or using an edge/fog network device. The services performed at this layer includes initialization, configuration, and synchronization of the sensors. Sensors readings are also collected at this layer for immediate processing and integration of data so as to provide real-time insight and decision making about the state of the user. The pregnant women could also be provided with audio and graphical interface to disseminating alert messages or needed guidance during medical crises. When the user is experiencing medical emergencies as indicated by the analyzed data, the Personal Server layer will establish a secured long-range Internet communication with the Medical Service layer and alert the respective remote healthcare service provider.

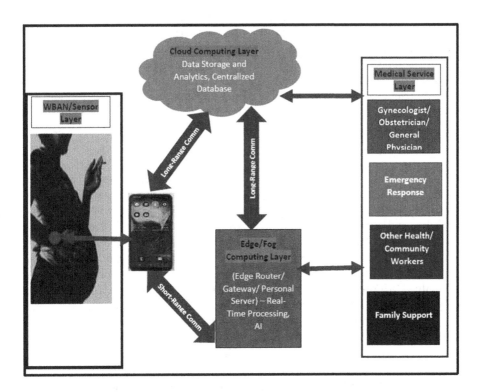

**Fig. 1.** Cloud-based IoT support for drug addicted pregnant women

### 5.3   Medical Service Layer

The Medical Service layer is made up of all the medical, family and community support services that are needed by pregnant women struggling with addiction. The layer allows real-time monitoring of the patient by service providers including Gynecologist, Obstetrician, General Physician, Emergency Response team, Health/Community Workers, families and friends. These groups of stakeholders are automatically contacted or alerted when there are cases of emergencies relating to the pregnant women (patient). Depending on the type of emergencies, the Personal Server layer will provide a detailed account of the situation of the patient, the current location of the patient and the level of support needed by the patient. In addition, the healthcare service providers will have access to a cloud-enabled centralized Medical Database that provides historical data and results of analysis of both current and previous data collected by the IoT system. The IoT system grants access to the centralized database depending on the level of services that are provided by a service provider. The advantages of the centralized Medical Database include providing real-time access to vital medical information about patients, providing deeper insights and decision making functionality based on the results of the Big Data analytics done in the cloud system, and preventing double-doctoring which can lead to multiple prescriptions of the same medication. Double-doctoring is a situation that can arise when there is no centralized medical database in which a doctor can prescribe a medication without reference to a previous prescription made by another doctor of the same medication. Also, the personal data collected through the sensors at the fog layer would be useful for medical personnels in providing swift medical support for COVID-19 infected pregnant women with underlying medical conditions.

### 5.4   Cloud Computing Layer

The physiological data collected overtime at the Personal Server layer can become so massive that it requires a larger, permanent and secured storage system. In addition, such Big Data requires a storage system where extensive processing and data analytics can be carried out so as to derive deeper insights into the patient's condition with the aim of proving decision making support for the medical practitioners. Therefore, the Cloud Computing layer serves as the center where the massive physiological data are aggregated, stored, processed and analyzed to provide support to healthcare service providers. The cloud system also hosts a centralized Medical Database where both historical and current medical data are stored for centralized access by medical practitioners and other healthcare stakeholders. As more and more data are being added from the Personal Server layer, machine learning algorithms could be engaged to allow the system to learn from the past and current data to make predictions and provide vital information about the patient's symptoms and possible diagnosis. Machine learning allows the identification of trends in medical physiological data that were formerly unidentified so as to provide specific diagnosis, treatment plans and decision support for healthcare service providers. The patients could also be alerted as a result of the outcome of the data analytics and machine learning algorithms implemented in the cloud. For instance, if the data collected suggests that a patient is becoming restless and agitated, the system could send an alert to the patient and instruct the patient on what can be done to calm down.

# 6 Big Data Problem in IoT Health Applications - A Case of Drug Addicted Women

The advent of IoT in health applications such as neonatal care and ambient assisted living [28], wellness recommendation [29], ECG health monitoring systems [30], and prognosis [31] accentuates the generation and collection of high volumes, high velocity, wide varieties, and valuable data with various degrees of veracity-popularly referred to as 5Vs of big data. Our proposed IoT and Data Analytics system for drug addicted women is made up of several sensors collecting vital data in different forms and format from users at real-time. The heterogeneous physiological data collected overtime from the users will gradually snowballed to a massive data. Some of the anticipated challenges of this Big Data collection from the IoT support system for the drug addicted women includes dealing with errors in the captured data, handling increase in time required for data processing and analytics, ensuring data privacy, and providing a scalable data storage system.

## 6.1 Data Analytics for IoT Health Support for Drug Addicted Pregnant Women

The Big Data collected from the addicted pregnant women would be a good platform for fine-grained data analytics that will provide deep insights on the pregnant women's health status. This platform can also provide intelligent recommendations for the physicians, emergency support unit, and other healthcare service providers. Therefore, the Data Analytics component of our proposed system will employ several data munging techniques such as feature extraction and dimensionality reduction to optimize the data and ensure that noise and redundancy are eliminated from the data. In addition, we will employ machine learning algorithms such as neural networks and decision trees to allow the system to learn from the past and current data for enhanced predictive analysis. This will help to provide vital information about the patient's symptoms and possible diagnosis. Besides, data mining techniques such as association rules would be employed to identify trends in medical physiological data that were formerly unidentified so as to provide specific diagnosis, treatment plans and decision support for healthcare service providers. We will ensure that a lightweight predictive algorithm is deployed at the Fog layer of our proposed IoT system so as to provide immediate and on-demand healthcare services to the users. Furthermore, our proposed system will profit from the implementation of Big Data processing frameworks including Apache Spark [32] and Kafka [33] so as to speed up the data analytics process and provide a platform for enhanced scalability as the size of the healthcare related data increases.

# 7   Conclusion and Future Research Direction

In this paper, we presented a non-invasive cloud-based IoT healthcare infrastructure for supporting pregnant women seeking treatments from drug misuse during pregnancy and public emergencies like COVID-19. We discovered that the current IoT systems that use bulky devices or devices inserted under the skin to monitor patients' vitals are not desirable in this application. The novelty of our proposed system stems from its ability to allow pregnant women seeking addiction treatment to continue with their normal daily activities while receiving intensive healthcare support without being confined to a facility. The system also profits from real-time local data analysis at the fog layer as well as the extensive data analysis at the cloud layer. The local data analysis provides immediate services to the pregnant women while the extensive cloud-based data analysis provides long term support for the pregnant women as well as the supporting health service providers. A detailed description of our Data Analytics approach will be presented in a future paper. In our future work, we plan to implement the IoT-based healthcare system with the aim of evaluating its efficiency and effectiveness in supporting the intended users. We will also consider relevant security and safety issues that have to do with the usage of the proposed system especially during global pandemics like COVID-19

# References

1. Baker, S.B., Xiang, W., Atkinson, I.: Internet of things for smart healthcare: technologies, challenges, and opportunities. IEEE Access **5**, 26521–26544 (2017)
2. Farahani, B., Firouzi, F., Chang, V., Badaroglu, M., Constant, N., Mankodiya, K.: Towards fog-driven IoT eHealth: promises and challenges of IoT in medicine and healthcare. Future Gener. Comput. Syst. **78**, 659–676 (2018)
3. Finnegan, L.: Substance abuse in Canada: licit and illicit drug use during pregnancy: Maternal, neonatal and early childhood consequences. Canadian Centre on Substance Abuse, Ottawa (2013)
4. Finnegan, L.P., Kandall, S.R.: Neonatal abstinence syndromes. In: Aranda, J., Jaffe, S.J. (eds.) Neonatal and Pediatric Pharmacology: Therapeutic Principles in Practice, 3rd edn. (2005)
5. Finnegan, L.P., Mellott, J.M., Ryan, L.M., Wapner, R.J.: Perinatal exposure to cocaine: human studies. In: Lakoski, J.M., Galloway, M.P., White, J. (eds.) Cocaine: Pharmacology, Physiology, and Clinical Strategies, pp. 391–409 (1992)
6. García-Valls, M., Calva-Urrego, C., García-Fornes, A.: Accelerating smart eHealth services execution at the fog computing infrastructure. Future Gener. Comput. Syst. (2018). https://doi.org/10.1016/j.future.2018.07.001
7. Health Canada: Canadian Alcohol and Drug Use Monitoring Survey: Summary of results for 2011 (2012)
8. Iqbal, M.M., Sobhan, T., Ryals, T.: Effects of commonly used benzodiazepines on the fetus, the neonate, and the nursing infant. Psychiatr. Serv. **53**(1), 39–49 (2002)
9. Kumari, A., Tanwar, S., Tyagi, S., Kumar, N.: Fog computing for Healthcare 4.0 environment: opportunities and challenges. Comput. Electr. Eng. **72**, 1–13 (2018)
10. Porath-Waller, A.J.: Clearing the smoke on cannabis: Maternal cannabis use during pregnancy. Canadian Centre on Substance Abuse, Ottawa (2009)

11. Poole, N.: Fetal Alcohol Spectrum Disorder (FASD) Prevention: Canadian Perspectives. Public Health Agency of Canada, Ottawa (2008)
12. Substance Abuse and Mental Health Services Administration (SAMHSA): Results from the 2010 National Survey on Drug Use and Health: Summary of national findings [NSDUH Series H-41, DHHS Publication No. SMA 11–4658]. Rockville, MD (2011)
13. Yang, Z., Zhou, Q., Lei, L., Zheng, K., Xiang, W.: An IoT-cloud based wearable ECG monitoring system for smart healthcare. J. Med. Syst. **40**, 286 (2016)
14. Dang, L.M., Piran, M.J., Han, D., Min, K., Moon, H.: A survey on internet of things and cloud computing for healthcare. Electronics **8**, 768–774 (2019)
15. National Institute of Drug Abuse (NIDA): The Science of Drug Use and Addiction: The Basics (2018). https://www.drugabuse.gov/publications/media-guide/science-drug-use-addiction-basics. Accessed 29 May 2020
16. O'Donoghue, J., Herbert, J. and Fensli, R. : Sensor Validation within a Pervasive Medical Environment. In: Proceedings of IEEE Sensors, South Korea (2006). ISBN 1-4244-0376-6
17. Pasluosta, C.F., Gassner, H., Winkler, J., Klucken, J., Eskofier, B.M.: An emerging era in the management of Parkinson's disease: wearable technologies and the internet of things. IEEE J. Biomed. Health Inf. **19**(6), 1873–1881 (2015)
18. Kaur, R.D.: Wireless body area network its application. Int. J. Eng. Sci. **1**, 199–216 (2011)
19. Abidi, B., Jilbab, A., Haziti, M.E.: Wireless sensor networks in biomedical: wireless body area networks. In: Rocha, Á., Serrhini, M., Felgueiras, C. (eds.) Europe and MENA Cooperation Advances in Information and Communication Technologies. Advances in Intelligent Systems and Computing, pp. 321–329. Springer, Heidelberg (2017)
20. Fan, Y.J., Yin, Y.H., Xu, L.D., Zeng, Y., Wu, F.: IoT based smart rehabilitation system. IEEE Trans. Ind. Inf. **10**(2), 1568–1577 (2014)
21. CFC Solutions: Unleash the Power of the Internet of Things, Cisco Systems Inc., San Jose (2015)
22. Sultan, N.: Making use of cloud computing for healthcare provision: opportunities and challenges. Int. J. Inf. Manag. **34**, 177–184 (2014)
23. Truong, H.L., Dustdar, S.: Principles for engineering IoT cloud systems. IEEE Cloud Comput. **2**, 68–76 (2015)
24. American Addiction Centers (AAC): Drug and Alcohol Withdrawal Symptoms, Timelines, and Treatment. (2015). https://americanaddictioncenters.org/withdrawal-timelines-treatments. Accessed 11 June 2020
25. Cretikos, M.A., Bellomo, R., Hillman, K., Chen, J., Finfer, S., Flabouris, A.: Respiratory rate: the neglected vital sign. Med. J. Aust. **188**, 657–659 (2008)
26. Center for Behavioral Health Statistics and Quality (CBHSQ): Key substance use and mental health indicators in the United States: Results from the 2015 National Survey on Drug Use and Health (HHS Publication No. SMA 16–4984, NSDUH Series H-51) (2016). Accessed 6 June 2020. https://www.samhsa.gov/data/
27. Florence, C.S., Zhou C., Luo F., Xu L.: The economic burden of prescription opioid overdose, abuse, and dependence in the United States, 2013. Med. Care. **54**(10):901-906 (2016). https://doi.org/10.1097/MLR.0000000000000625
28. Arijit, M., Arpan, P., Prateep, M.: Data analytics in ubiquitous sensor-based health information systems. In: Proceedings of the 6th International Conference on Next Generation Mobile Applications, Services, and Technologies (2012). https://doi.org/10.1109/NGMAST.2012.39

29. Oresti, B., et al.: The mining minds digital health and wellness framework. Biomed. Eng. **76** (2016). https://doi.org/10.1186/s12938-016-0179-9
30. Hossain, M.S., Muhammad, G.: Cloud-assisted industrial internet of things (IIoT) - enabled framework for health monitoring. Comput. Netw. **101**, 192–202 (2015). https://doi.org/10.1016/j.comnet.2016.01.009
31. Myriam, H., et al.: Decision making in health and medicine: integrating evidence and values. Cambridge University Press, London (2014). http://jrsm.rsmjournals.com/cgi/doi/10.1258/jrsm.95.2.108-a
32. Sarumi, O.A., Leung, C.K., Adetunmbi, A.O.: Spark-based data analytics of sequence motifs in large omics data. Procedia Comput. Sci. **126**, 596–605 (2018)
33. Le Noac'h, P., Costan, A., Boug e, L. : A performance evaluation of Apache Kafka in support of big data streaming applications. In: IEEE International Conference on Big Data (Big Data), pp. 4803–4806 (2017)
34. Ignite, IoT: Android as a Gateway (2020). https://devzone.iot-ignite.com/knowledge-base/android-as-a-gateway/. Accessed 14 June 2020

# Sensors Characterization for a Calibration-Free Connected Smart Insole for Healthy Ageing

Luca Gioacchini[1] , Angelica Poli[2] , Stefania Cecchi[2] ,
and Susanna Spinsante[2(✉)]

[1] Department of Electronics and Telecommunications, Politecnico di Torino,
10129 Turin, Italy
s257076@studenti.polito.it
[2] Department of Information Engineering, Università Politecnica delle Marche,
60131 Ancona, Italy
{a.poli,s.cecchi,s.spinsante}@staff.univpm.it

**Abstract.** The design of technological aids to assist older adults in their ageing process and to ensure proper attendance and care, despite the decreasing percentage of young people in the demographic profiles of many developed countries, requires the proper selection of sensing components, in order to come up with devices that can be easily used and integrated into everyday life. This paper addresses the metrological characterization of pressure sensors to be inserted into smart insoles aimed at monitoring the older adult's physical activity levels. Two types of sensing elements are evaluated and a recommendation provided, based on the main requirement of designing a calibration-free insole: in this case, the pressure sensor should act as a switch, and the FSR 402 Short sensing element appears to be the proper solution to adopt.

**Keywords:** Smart insole · Force Sensing Resistor · Step counter · Healthy ageing

## 1 Introduction

In the last years, world population has undergone a demographic transition, in which the mortality and the birth rates both decreased. This means that globally, world population is shifting from a young age structure towards an old age one. The number of elders, especially in developed and wealthy countries, has increased and is now 10% higher than the number of young people. Because of the illnesses that

Supported by the Europen Union's Active Assisted Living Programme under grant agreement AAL2017-63-vINCI, and the Italian Ministero dell'Istruzione, Università e Ricerca (CUP: I34I17000010005) within the project *vINCI*: "Clinically-validated INtegrated Support for Assistive Care and Lifestyle Improvement: the Human Link" (https://vinci.ici.ro/). Authors wish to thank the project partner Optima Molliter Srl for the provisioning of test devices.

© ICST Institute for Computer Sciences, Social Informatics and Telecommunications Engineering 2021
Published by Springer Nature Switzerland AG 2021. All Rights Reserved
R. Goleva et al. (Eds.): HealthyIoT 2020, LNICST 360, pp. 35–54, 2021.
https://doi.org/10.1007/978-3-030-69963-5_3

inevitably appear after a certain age, or simply because the physical resources dry out as people grow old, at some point older adults may find themselves in need for attendance and caring. But, due to the demographic ageing, there are fewer and fewer young people who can assist the older ones. This is the reason why there is a great need for an extra helping hand, something that can *aid both the elderly and the people who take care of them.* This huge help can be achieved through so called *assistive technology* (AT).

Research projects like vINCI [12] address the situation, aiming at designing the technological support that the elders and their caregivers need. Its purpose is to integrate different devices needed to monitor and improve the older adult's life, in a single, unifying platform. Moreover, it targets to enhance and sustain active aging of older adults, with devices like smart watches, smart insoles, monitoring cameras, together with tablets and properly designed software applications, which can be differently combined and composed according to the user's needs and preferences. In order to reach these goals, certain technical requirements must be met, either at the device and the cloud platform level. Not only devices must be able to connect to the platform and send data in a proper and recognized format, but also the cloud needs to be available all the time to prevent any data loss and to satisfy the users that interact with the dashboards or applications. All the interfaces need to be user-friendly and intuitive, especially because the users consists of older people who can be not very familiar with technology.

Among the requirements pertaining to the devices connected to the monitoring platform, a specific one refers to smart insoles [1], like those shown in Fig. 1. These are wearable devices, connected over a Bluetooth Low Energy (BLE) link to a smartphone or eventually equipped with a long-range communication interface [10], which can be easily inserted into a user's common shoes, and they allow to count the steps performed in a day, and to recognize different motion statuses, such as walking, standing, sitting or not wearing the insole [5,11]. According to the World Health Organization (WHO) guidelines about physical activity (PA)

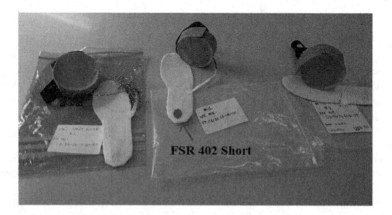

**Fig. 1.** Smart insoles prototypes developed within the vINCI project.

in the older age [9], the amount of steps performed by an older adult in a day is a very important indicator of their physical and mental health status [6, 7]. In order to have devices that can be easily used by older adults, without the need for complex calibration processes, like those typically requested by smart insoles designed for sport and fitness purposes, a calibration-free design must be targeted. In fact, we aim for a device which is not expected to estimate the walked distance or the amount of burnt calories but, surprisingly, such a smart insole is currently not available in the market. As a consequence, this paper addresses the technical design of the smart insoles, specifically focusing on the proper selection of the sensing elements, which should allow to fulfill the expected aims avoiding the need for calibrating the subject's walking profile. The main contribution of this paper is the metrological characterization of two different types of pressure sensors, in order to identify the most suitable solution for the design of a durable smart insole able to provide reliable data about the user's PA, despite not requiring the calibration of the device by the user.

The paper is organized as follows: Sect. 2 shortly reviews the state-of-the-art about sensorized insoles for physical activity monitoring. Section 3 presents the design of the sensing insole, including motivations and sensors selection. Materials and methods for sensors characterization are presented in Sect. 4, while Sect. 5 presents and discusses the results obtained, under different conditions and analyses. Finally, Sect. 6 concludes the paper.

## 2   Background

Looking at the recent results about the design of smart insoles and in-shoe sensor systems, it appears that most of the studies are aimed at specific applications with clinical outcomes, such as gait analysis, real-time estimation of temporal gait parameters, foot motion analysis, and health monitoring.

Tahir et al. [13] discuss the growing interest in developing smart insoles associated to gait analysis, to be exploited in rehabilitation, clinical diagnostics and sport activities applications. Specifically, vertical Ground Reaction Forces (vGRF) and other gait variables could be measured by suitably designed wearable devices, able to continuously monitor plantar pressure through embedded sensors converting it into an electrical signal that can be further processed and eventually transmitted. In applications having potential clinical impact, it is important to use calibrated sensors to provide reliable measurements. In the mentioned work, authors state that calibration approaches adopted by different teams required expensive instruments such as universal testing machines or infrared motion capture cameras. In contrast, authors propose a systematic design and characterization procedure for three different types of pressure sensors: force-sensitive resistors (FSRs), ceramic piezoelectric sensors, and flexible piezoelectric sensors that can be used for detecting vGRF in a smart insole. The FSR proves to be the most effective sensor among the three tested, for smart insole applications. Shoe-embedded sensors have potentially huge advantages for the design of wearable robotic devices aimed at locomotion-related applications.

In [3], the development of a pair of pressure-sensitive insoles based on opto-electronic sensors for the real-time estimation of temporal gait parameters is presented. The system is assessed relatively to both vGRF and progression, providing satisfactory results in tests of ground-level walking at two speeds involving ten healthy participants. Recent advances in research concerning smart socks and in-shoe systems for foot motion analysis and health monitoring are reviewed in [2]. The considered devices represent textile-based systems and pressure sensitive insole (PSI) systems, respectively. They are analyzed with respect to special medical applications, for gait and foot pressure analysis, in comparison to the Pedar system used in medicine and sports. This paper aims to provide readers with a detailed overview of the above mentioned devices, to possibly improve their design and functionality, and find new application areas.

Considering the design of a connected smart insole for healthy aging-related applications, previous papers from some of the co-authors [1,5,10,11] mostly addressed the electronics components and the data transmission interface. In this paper, the focus is on the choice and characterization of the sensing elements to be inserted into the insole, targeting a calibration-free device. With respect to the state-of-the-art presented above and summarized in Table 1, the current work provides details about the behavior of two specific pressure sensors selected for a smart insole not aimed at clinical observation but at the monitoring of PA in older adults. Usability and avoidance of complex configuration procedures are the leading design criteria for the device.

**Table 1.** Summary of recent smart insoles development in the literature.

| Research paper | Application and main results |
| --- | --- |
| Tahir et al. [13] | Wearable sensors employed to detect vertical ground reaction forces (vGRF) and other gait variables. The paper provides a systematic design and characterization procedure for three different pressure sensors: FSRs, ceramic piezoelectric sensors, and flexible piezoelectric sensors |
| Martini et al. [3] | The development of a pair of pressure-sensitive insoles based on optoelectronic sensors for the real-time estimation of temporal gait parameters is presented |
| Dragulinescu et al. [2] | Both textile-based and pressure sensitive insole (PSI) systems are analyzed with respect to special medical applications, for gait and foot pressure analysis |

## 3 Design of the Sensing Insole

### 3.1 Motivations

The decision to address the design of a smart insole for the aims of the vINCI project purposes, was motivated by the fact that, performing a deep and careful analysis of the devices available in the market, a few potential candidates were found, which were however not suitable for the project.

As a matter of fact, commercial devices such as Digitsole smart insole (https://www.digitsole.com/) or Moticon sensor insole (https://www.moticon.de/) are designed for runners and people interested in monitoring their performances during physical activities. In order to do so and to estimate, among others, the distance covered during a run or in general during the whole day just by walking, these devices typically require a *calibration procedure* with the user running on a treadmill, at different paces, for specific amount of time. For example, in the case of the insoles sold by Digitsole, the user is recommended to take about 200 steps at a fast pace so that the soles can analyze how he/she runs. The calibration shall be completed for a more detailed analysis of the strokes, as it allows the insoles to better understand the runner profile and therefore to more effectively measure the subsequent performance. Such a calibration, joint with details about height, weight, gender and age of the subject, provided through a specific app designed on purpose for the device, also enables the estimation of the amount of calories burnt by a subject, over a given period of time. It would not be possible for many older adults to perform such a type of calibration process. In general, this could be a barrier to the use of the smart insole by older customers, as addressed by the project.

For these reasons, we aimed at designing a smart insole that can enable the unobtrusive monitoring of the physical activity performed by an older adult, without requiring a calibration process. Of course, this choice implies that some functionalities, such as the estimation of the walked distance and the amount of calories burnt will not be possible. However, taking into account the fact that PA in older adults is defined in a broader way than for younger subjects (consider, for example, the definition of *light activity* [14] by the National Health System in UK), the design of the device can be somehow simplified and made more acceptable by users. Specifically, the design was based on the use of Force Sensing Resistors (FSRs) as pressure transducers, to generate signals from which both the number of steps performed and the type of PA carried out can be attained. Accelerometers are not considered in a first design phase, aiming for the simplest data processing possible, leading to minimal hardware requirements.

## 3.2   Sensors Selection

Two kinds of sensors were evaluated to identify the viable solution: the FSR 402 Short provided by Interlink Electronics, and the FlexiForce A301 provided by Tekscan.

**FSR 402 Short.** This tiny device, based on the thick-film technology, is basically a resistor which allows to detect weight and pressure by changing its resistance value. The use of this sensor model is suggested for the majority of do-it-yourself (DIY) Arduino-based projects and applications. The sensor essential design shown in Fig. 2(a) consists of two layers separated by a spacer.

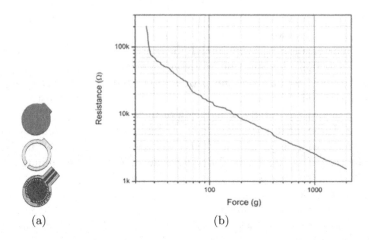

Fig. 2. (a) FSR 402 Short design. (b) FSR 402 Short Resistance/Force curve.

The upper layer (called FSR layer) is made of some flexible material such as PET or polymide, coated with FSR carbon-based ink. The spacer has the double function of keeping together the two layers and maintaining the air gap. Its thickness is between 0.03 mm ad 0.15 mm. The lower layer consists of a flexible polymer sheet such as polycarbonate or thin metal. It has also two sets of inter-digited traces. When the user applies a pressure on the bottom layer, the FSR ink shorts with the two tracks generating a variable resistance. The advantage of this technology is the increased miniaturization of the sensor provided by the incorporation of the passive element into the substrate. It allows a wide range of resistance with reasonable curing temperature, even if the resistance value becomes more unstable over the long period (especially with high temperature and humidity conditions). Interlink Electronics states that the force sensitivity range goes from 0.2 N to 20 N with a minimum of 0.2 N as actuation force. By using a repeatable actuation system, the repeatability of the single part is about $\pm 2\%$ of the initial reading. The long term drift ensured is $<5\%$ per $\log_{10}$ (time). This data is referred to 35 days of testing with 1 kg load. The hysteresis is $+10\%$ of the full scale. In Fig. 2(b) the sensor resistance trend is shown, when the applied force changes. The actuation force is the one required to bring the sensor from the open circuit condition to below 100 k$\Omega$ resistance.

**FlexiForce A301.** Tekscan provides these piezoresistive sensors whose behavior is determined by *strain* and the *Hooke's Law*. The former is defined as the relative change in the shape or size of an elastic object due to an applied force. The latter states that the strain of an elastic object is directly proportional to the applied force. This way, it is clear that by measuring the physical changing of an object after the application of a force it is possible to measure the force itself. The most common device used for this purpose is an electrical resistance strain gauge, since the resistance of a conductor is directly proportional to its length and inversely

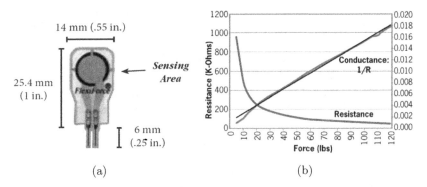

**Fig. 3.** (a) FlexiForce A301 design. (b) Resistance/Force and Conductance/Force trends for a 100lb FlexiForce A301 sensor (in black, an ideal linear dependency between force and output resistance).

proportional to its cross-sectional area:

$$R = \int_{\Delta L} \frac{\rho(l)dl}{S(l)} \tag{1}$$

where $\rho(l)$ is the electrical resistivity of the conductor, $S(l)$ is the cross sectional area and $\Delta L$ is the length variation of the conductor. If the resistance is attached to an elastic element, when it is modified, the resistance length changes too. As we can see in Fig. 3(b) the resistance has a non-linear trend with strain, so usually a linearization circuit is required.

Having clarified the basic principles, we have to consider that the A301 is made of a piezoresistive material located between two conductive layers. This particular material differs from a simply resistive one from the fact that its resistance depends on the force applied to the material, rather than its size change. Similar to the FSR sensor, the resistance of a piezoresistive one drops from several MΩ when no force is applied, to a few kΩ when pressed.

Tekscan provides three versions of this sensor: the first one can tolerate a maximum 4.4 N load, the second one a 111 N load, and the third one a 445 N load. By using a repeatable actuation system, the ensured repeatability is ±2.5% of the initial reading. The long term drift ensured is <5% per $\log_{10}$(time), tested with a constant 111 N load. The hysteresis is <4.5% of the full scale.

## 4   Materials and Method for Sensors Characterization

The measurement setup for sensor characterization is presented in this section. It consists of an Arduino UNO board with a voltage divider, a baropodometric platform and a software tool developed in Python to control the Arduino board, and allow the serial communication with the computer. Two main functions are implemented: the former enables the acquisition of a single resistance value and it is used for a preliminary check of operation. The latter allows a continuous stream of data and plots them. The acquisition is stopped manually by the operator.

The role of the Arduino board is to acquire the variations of the sensor resistance originated by the pressure applied on it. Sensors are connected to the board through a voltage divider shown in Fig. 4, where the variable resistance $R_2$ represents the sensor, whereas $R_1$ is a reference resistance of fixed value. This way, the variation of resistance is converted into a voltage signal to measure, named $V_{out}$, which is given by:

$$V_{out} = V_{in} \frac{R_2}{R_1 + R_2} \tag{2}$$

The reference voltage $V_{in}$ is 5 V and it is taken directly from one of the Arduino pin. The $V_{out}$ value is taken from an analog reading of the A0 pin of the board. The Arduino sampling frequency 20 Hz and the ADC (Analog to Digital Converter) has a resolution of 10 bits. In order to get the sensor resistance value, the following equations are applied:

$$R_{sensor} = \frac{V_{in} - V_{out}}{V_{out}} \cdot R_1 \tag{3}$$

$$V_{out} = \frac{V_{in} \cdot V_{read}}{1024} \tag{4}$$

Where $R_{sensor}$ is the resistance value of the sensor, $V_{read}$ is the analog read voltage (it must be converted according to the Arduino ADC resolution: a 10-bit resolution involves a range of 1024 values), $V_{out}$ is the real output tension and $R_1$ is the 10 k$\Omega$ reference resistance.

A fixed dynamometric platform (Bertec H4060) based on strain gauge technology is used as the reference measurement instrument [4], in such a way to have a calibrated and accurate measurement of the force applied on the sensor. Data from the platform are acquired by means of a professional movement analysis system (Elite, BTS-Bioengineering, Italy) with a sampling rate 500 Hz.

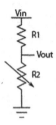

**Fig. 4.** Voltage divider used for the sensors characterization.

Two different experiment sessions were carried out: the former with heavy weights, the latter with light weights. Since we want to characterize force sensitive resistors, we need to known exactly how heavy is the applied load, and its distribution over the measuring devices. So, we used a 3 kg triangular medium shown in Fig. 5 as a supporting tool to measure heavy weights, and a 0.6 kg wooden medium to help measuring light weights. Both of them were based on three rebars slightly smaller than the sensors sensitive areas. This way, by adding loads over the medium, we can be sure that the weight is evenly distributed on the sensor active area. The load consists of an increasing number of 10 kg and 1 kg weight plates for the first kind of data acquisitions, and an increasing number of 0.1 kg of water-filled elements in the range [0.1, 0.3] kg for the second one.

In order to get an accurate measurement of the force (in Newton) applied on the sensor we used the baropodometric platform (shown in Fig. 5) for the high weights measurements and an electronic kitchen scale with resolution 1 g for the low weights ones. This way it is possible to determine the resistance value in relation to the applied force. It is important to explain the measurement procedure when the baropodometric platform is used: at the beginning of each measurement, it is necessary to clear out the platform in order to measure the no-load offset. After that, the operator can put the load and start the measurement. Since Arduino and the force platform are stand-alone devices, as shown in Fig. 6, the trigger for their synchronisation was verbally determined by two computer operators. The output of the takes is a pair of .dat files ready to be processed. Because of the different

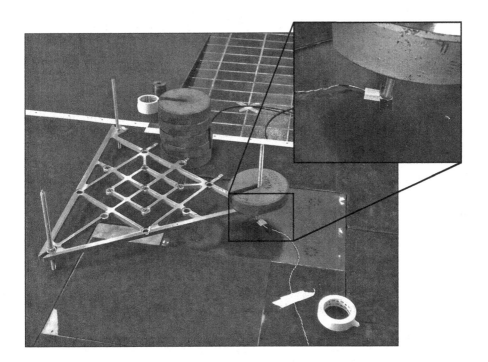

**Fig. 5.** Experimental measurement setup.

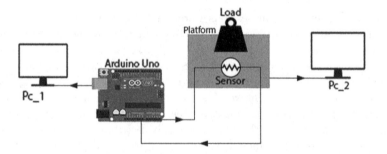

**Fig. 6.** Functional scheme of the measurement setup.

sampling frequencies of the two devices and the approximate vocal trigger for the acquisition, data should be downsampled 20 Hz and the excess values should be discarded, to obtain a matrix without zeros.

## 5   Experimental Results and Discussion

In this section the experimental results about mean resistance values measurements are presented, as well as considerations relating to the drift phenomenon affecting the sensors under evaluation.

### 5.1   Sensors Characterization in the Case of High Weights

**Mean Resistance/Force (R/F) Values.** Some first useful measurements are obtained as the mean values of the resistance assumed by the sensors during each measurement operation[1].

In Fig. 7 and Fig. 8 the trend of the resistance values assumed by the FSR 402 Short and the relative scatter-plots obtained during two measurement sessions are reported. In Fig. 9 and Fig. 10 the same results are shown when the FlexiForce A301 is used.

As we can see from the plots in Fig. 7 and Fig. 9, by applying the 3 kg medium only on the sensors (i.e. performing an off-load measurement), none of them reaches the saturation condition, even if the FSR assumes a resistance value much lower than the FlexiForce one (0.68 kΩ compared with 225.58 kΩ).

By applying a load of about 13 kg[2] on the devices, a different behavior of the sensors is observed. The 402 Short sensor enters its saturation zone: it takes on a 0.21 kΩ resistance value from which the following variations are very small, even when increasing the applied load. In fact, by adding an increased amount of weight, the measured resistance decreases a little, down to a *floor* of about 0.16 kΩ. On the other hand, the A301 sensor, whose datasheet ensures a maximum

---

[1] E.g. three consecutive measurement operations are performed, by applying 12 N on the sensor, so the values plotted in Fig. 7 are the mean of each measurement session.

[2] 10 kg weight plate plus 3 kg of the supporting medium.

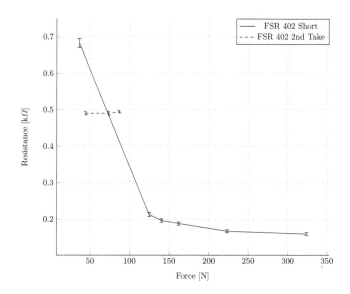

**Fig. 7.** FSR 402 Short force/resistance trend. Plotted values are the mean ones collected during the acquisitions. It is indicated the standard deviation of each value. The dashed line shows the resistance values obtained when 4.5 kg, 7.5 kg and 8.9 kg are applied in a second measurement session.

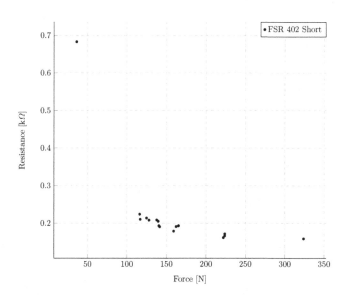

**Fig. 8.** Force/resistance values scatter plot of the FSR 402 Short sensor for the same applied load values of Fig. 7.

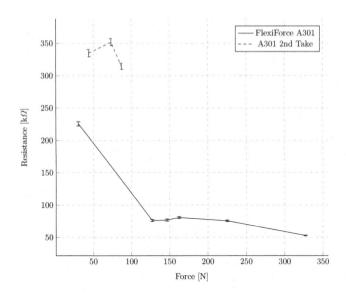

**Fig. 9.** FlexiForce A301 force/resistance trend. Plotted values are the mean ones collected during the acquisitions. It is indicated the standard deviation of each value. The dashed line shows the resistance values obtained when 4.5 kg, 7.5 kg and 8.9 kg load values are applied in a second measurement session.

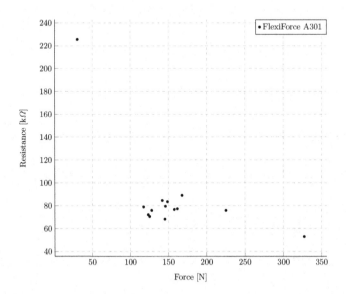

**Fig. 10.** Force/resistance values scatter plot of the FlexiForce A301 sensor for the same applied load values of Fig. 9.

load of 45 kg, is still in its linear working zone. As we can see from Fig. 9, the R/F curve keeps a slight concavity and a little offset corresponding to the [13] kg range. This means that the range of values assumed by the sensor is still wide, and not limited by the floor resistance value (by applying a 146.6 N load, a resistance value of 76.9 kΩ is obtained; for a 327.18 N load, the resistance value is 52.8 kΩ). This is also confirmed by Fig. 8, in which the value markers of each measurement are densely placed around the floor resistance value, while in Fig. 10 they are more widespread.

The dashed lines of Fig. 7 and Fig. 9 show the resistance values assumed by the FSR 402 Short and the FlexiForce A301 sensors, respectively, when 4.5 kg, 7.5 kg and 8.9 kg are applied, during a different measurement session. Even if the resistance values exhibited by the 402 Short sensor are not representative of the general trend obtained during the first test, they lie within a range of values coherent with the other measurements. On the other hand, the resistance values provided by the A301 sensor are quite patchy. We can assume that this is because for this different measurement session we used a commercial balance, which is not so sensitive to the 0.1-fold weight variations. Furthermore, we changed the specific sensor devices under test (even if, of course, belonging to the same FSR 402 Short and FlexiForce A301 families). This means that each sensor item is more or less sensible to weight variations, so it would always request an a priori calibration, if aimed at *measuring* the force value applied. We need also to observe the position of the supporting medium on the sensors' active areas. In fact, if the medium is barely located on the A301 spacer, this can affect the weight distribution, causing a possible resistance value shift of up to 100 kΩ.

**Drift Evaluation.** Another useful data for a sensor characterization is the drift factor. Considering the procedures used in [8], the drift analysis has been led through a 60 s-long static measurement when the sensors are in their linear working zone, so when the 3 kg medium only is applied on the FSR 402 Short, and when a 20 kg-weight plate plus the 3 kg medium is located on the A301 sensor. Measuring the initial and final value of the resistance, given by $R_i$ and $R_f$, respectively, the percent drift of the resistance value ($D_R$) is calculated as:

$$D_R = 100 \cdot (R_f - R_i)/R_i \tag{5}$$

Figure 11 and Fig. 12 provide a qualitative information about the sensors' drift reporting the resistance values oscillations and decreasing exhibited by the sensors during the constant weight application.

Even if the A301 resistance floats over a greater number of different values, after 60 s (i.e. 1200 samples), the drift factor is about the 6.94% of the initial value. This is lower than the FSR 402 Short one, which is about the 10% of the initial value, as shown in Fig. 11.

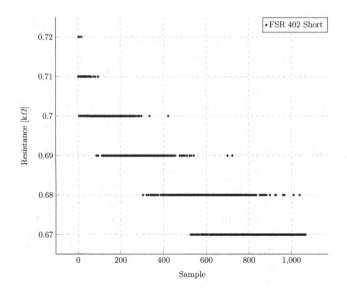

**Fig. 11.** Scatter plot of the FSR 402 Short sensor when the 3 kg medium is statically applied for a time of 60 s, aimed at its drift analysis.

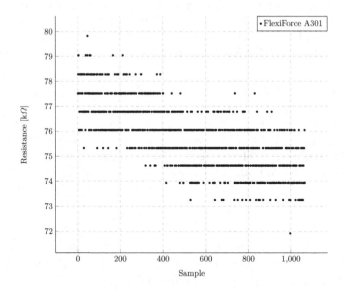

**Fig. 12.** Scatter plot of the FlexiForce A301 sensor when the 23 kg are applied for 60 s for a drift analysis.

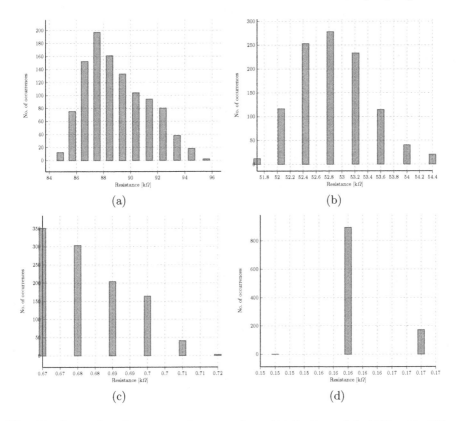

**Fig. 13.** Comparison between resistance values distributions: (a) A301 with 23 kg applied, linear working zone; (b) A301 with 33 kg applied, linear working zone, but near to the saturation one; (c) 402 Short with 3 kg applied, linear working zone, but near to the saturation one; (d) 402 Short with 13 kg applied, entering the saturation working zone.

By considering that both datasheets ensured a drift factor <5% of the initial value, it is clear that the FlexiForce sensor is not so far from this condition, while the FSR one has a quite different performance. Another consideration is necessary. By calculating the mean drift factor of all the acquisition takes for each sensor, it results that the 402 Short sensor has a drift factor equal to the 3.33% of the initial value, while the A301 one is about the 5.22% of the initial values. This results seem to conflict with all the previous considerations. However it should be noticed that during most of the measurements the FSR worked in its saturation zone, so, as far as a constant weight is applied, its resistance value cannot be lower than the floor one. Therefore, it is clear that the drift factor will certainly be lower than the A301 one, which works in linear zone and can assume a wider range of value.

To investigate the distributions of the resistance values assumed by the sensors, Fig. 13 show the values frequency of the A301 and FSR 402 in linear working zone and when the saturation one is approached. In all the cases, by gradually approaching the saturation working zone, the amount of values the sensors' resistance can assume decreases. When the weight applied on the A301 is 23 kg, the sensor resistance floats among 12 values (Fig. 13(a)). In Fig. 13(b) the weight applied is about 33 kg. By remembering that the maximum admitted weight for this sensor is 45 kg, we are approaching the saturation working zone, so the number of values assumed by the resistance goes down to 8. By applying about 3 kg on the FSR 402 sensor (Fig. 13(c)), we are in a border working zone, so the number of assumed resistance values is 6. When a 13 kg weight it is applied on it (Fig. 13(d)), this number decreases even further, to 3 values, floating around the floor. In view of this, data is consistent with what has been observed before.

### 5.2   Sensors Characterization in the Case of Low Weights

Very different results are obtained from the low weights measurements as it can be seen from the trend and scatter plot of Fig. 14 and Fig. 15 for the FSR 402. In this case the sensors exhibit a reverse behaviour: the FSR 402 Short seems to be more sensitive to the 0.1-fold weight variations. As it is shown in Fig. 14 and Fig. 15, except for a little offset when 2.1 kg and 2.2 kg are applied, the Force/Resistance trend is more akin to the datasheet one, and the standard

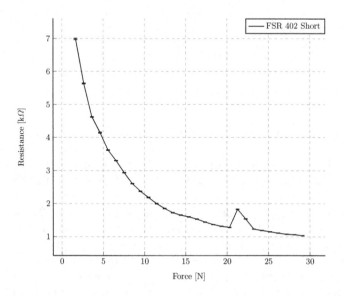

**Fig. 14.** Low weight FSR 402 Short Force/Resistance trend. Plotted values are the mean ones collected during the acquisitions. The standard deviation of each value is also reported.

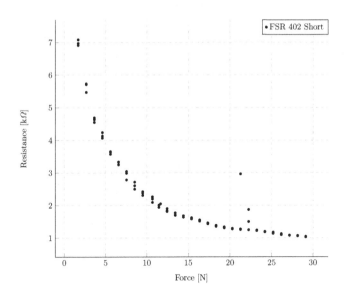

**Fig. 15.** Low weights Force/Resistance values scatter plot of the FSR 402 Short sensor.

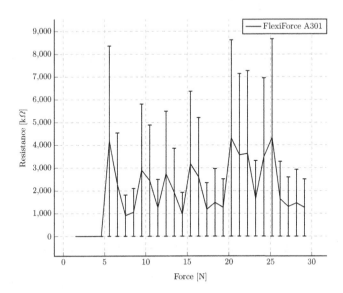

**Fig. 16.** Low weight FlexiForce A301 Force/Resistance trend. Plotted values are the mean ones collected during the acquisitions. The standard deviation of each value is also reported.

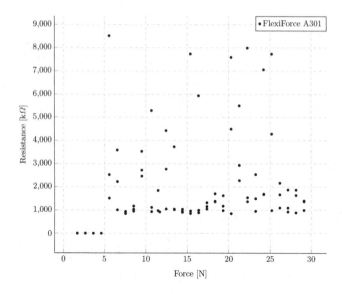

**Fig. 17.** Low weights Force/Resistance values scatter plot of the FlexiForce A301 sensor.

deviation is very small, so the resistance values are quite accurate. Furthermore, when 2.9 kg are applied on the sensor, its resistance value is about 1.032 k$\Omega$, which, according to what we have said at the end of Sect. 5.1, after a previous calibration, should be easily led to 0.68 k$\Omega$ of the Fig. 7. By observing the plots in Fig. 16 and Fig. 17, in which the resistance values trend and scatter plot for the FlexiForce are reported, it is clear that the A301 sensor is not very sensitive to low weights variations. In fact, it does not work until 0.5 kg are applied on it. After that threshold, the resistance values don't have an identifiable pattern and the standard deviation values are greater than in the other cases. This means that after 30 s of acquisition, the resistance values float between a certain value and zero. We can explain this behaviour by the fact that the activation force of this sensor has not been reached yet, and so, over the long term, it exhibits an unstable output.

## 6   Conclusion

Following the results presented above, two kinds of applications may be targeted by the examined sensors: those exploiting the sensor as a switch, and those which use it as an indicator of the weight applied. The specific devices tested may be recommended for the first kind of applications. In fact, after having selected a certain threshold, based on the calibration results performed in the lab on each sensor item, the random floating of the attained resistance values becomes irrelevant to the application. Then, the sensor to use should be selected based on the expected load and the supported range. As far as the second kind of application is concerned, A301 sensors are recommended for high weights and the FSR 402 Short for the low ones, especially for touch-based interaction applications, thanks to the high sensitivity of the device. Based on these findings, the FSR used in the first insole prototype design was the FSR 402 Short, to detect, by means of a proper software application running on the embedded board, the three different activity statuses mentioned before. The raw sensor measurements are not transmitted; the information about the status is generated onboard, by processing locally the raw sensor measurements. Transmissions from the insole take place only at a status change, and whenever the step counter increases. As a future development of the smart insole design, it is foreseen to integrate the FSR data with acceleration measurements, in order to improve the PA detection, the classification of the activity performed, and, possibly, to implement the evaluation of the covered distance within a day.

**Acknowledgment.** Authors wish to thank Dr. Federica Verdini from the Information Engineering Department at the Marche Polytechnic University for her help in collecting measurements from the baropodometric platform available at the Movement Analysis Bioengineering Lab.

# References

1. De Santis, A., Gambi, E., Montanini, L., Raffaeli, L., Spinsante, S., Rascioni, G.: A simple object for elderly vitality monitoring: the smart insole. In: 2014 IEEE/ASME 10th International Conference on Mechatronic and Embedded Systems and Applications (MESA), pp. 1–6 (2014)
2. Drăgulinescu, A., Drăgulinescu, A.M., Zincă, G., Bucur, D., Feie, V., Neagu, D.M.: Smart socks and in-shoe systems: state-of-the-art for two popular technologies for foot motion analysis, sports, and medical applications. Sensors **20**(15) (2020). https://doi.org/10.3390/s20154316. https://www.mdpi.com/1424-8220/20/15/4316
3. Martini, E., et al.: Pressure-sensitive insoles for real-time gait-related applications. Sensors **20**(5) (2020). https://doi.org/10.3390/s20051448. https://www.mdpi.com/1424-8220/20/5/1448
4. Mengarelli, A., Cardarelli, S., Tigrini, A., Fioretti, S., Verdini, F.: Kinetic data simultaneously acquired from dynamometric force plate and Nintendo Wii Balance Board during human static posture trials. Data Brief **28**, 105028 (2020). https://doi.org/10.1016/j.dib.2019.105028. http://www.sciencedirect.com/science/article/pii/S2352340919313848
5. Montanini, L., Del Campo, A., Perla, D., Spinsante, S., Gambi, E.: A footwear-based methodology for fall detection. IEEE Sens. J. **18**(3), 1233–1242 (2018). https://doi.org/10.1109/JSEN.2017.2778742
6. Mura, G., Mauro Giovanni, C.: Physical activity in depressed elderly. A systematic review. Clin. Pract. Epidemiol. Mental Health **9**, 125–135 (2013)
7. Nakamura, Y., Tanaka, K., Yabushita, N., Sakai, T., Shigematsu, R.: Effects of exercise frequency on functional fitness in older adult women. Arch. Gerontol. Geriatr. **44**(2), 163–173 (2007)

8. Parmar, S., Khodasevych, I., Troynikov, O.: Evaluation of flexible force sensors for pressure monitoring in treatment of chronic venous disorders. Sensors **17**(8) (2017). https://doi.org/10.3390/s17081923. https://www.mdpi.com/1424-8220/17/8/1923

9. Physical Activity Guidelines Advisory Committee (PAGAC): Physical activity guidelines advisory committee report (2018). https://www.who.int/dietphysicalactivity/factsheet_olderadults/en/. Accessed 03 Oct 2020

10. Spinsante, S., Poli, A., Pirani, S., Gioacchini, L.: Lora evaluation in mobility conditions for a connected smart shoe measuring physical activity. In: 2019 IEEE International Symposium on Measurements Networking (M N), pp. 1–5 (2019)

11. Spinsante, S., Scalise, L.: Measurement of elderly daily physical activity by unobtrusive instrumented shoes. In: 2018 IEEE International Symposium on Medical Measurements and Applications (MeMeA), pp. 1–5 (2018)

12. Spinsante, S., et al.: Integrated consumer technologies for older adults' quality of life improvement: the vINCI project. In: 2019 IEEE 23rd International Symposium on Consumer Technologies (ISCT), pp. 273–278 (2019)

13. Tahir, A.M., et al.: A systematic approach to the design and characterization of a smart insole for detecting vertical ground reaction force (vGRF) in gait analysis. Sensors **20**(4) (2020). https://doi.org/10.3390/s20040957. https://www.mdpi.com/1424-8220/20/4/957

14. UK National Health System: Physical activity guidelines for older adults. https://www.nhs.uk/live-well/exercise/physical-activity-guidelines-older-adults/. Accessed 11 Sept 2020

# Novel Wearable System for Surface EMG Using Compact Electronic Board and Printed Matrix of Electrodes

Tiziano Fapanni$^{(\boxtimes)}$ ⓘ, Nicola Francesco Lopomo ⓘ, Emilio Sardini ⓘ, and Mauro Serpelloni ⓘ

Department of Information Engineering, University of Brescia, Brescia, Italy
{t.fapanni,nicola.lopomo,emilio.sardini,
mauro.serpelloni}@unibs.it

**Abstract.** In recent years, the application of IoT for health purposes, including the intense use of wearable devices, has been considerably growing. Among the wearable devices, the systems for measuring EMG (electromyography) signals are highly investigated. The possibility of recording different signals in a multi-channel approach can lead to reliable data that can be used to improve diagnostic techniques, analyze performance in sports professionals and perform remote rehabilitation. In this work, we describe the design of a novel wearable system for surface EMG using a compact electronic board and a printed matrix of electrodes. The whole system has an estimated maximum current absorption of 55 mA at 3.3 V. We focused on the subsystem integration and on the real-time data transmission through Bluetooth Low Energy (BLE) with a throughput of 28 kB/s with a success rate of 99%. Some preliminary data are collected on a healthy man's arm to validate the design. The acquired data are then analyzed and processed to improve information quality and extract contraction patterns.

**Keywords:** Multielectrode EMG · Wearable device · Printed electrodes

## 1 Introduction

In the last decades, the measurement of physiological signals from the human body has raised great interest to the scientific community, as it allows monitoring subjects' health [1], diagnosing diseases, and providing suitable therapies [2] also for rehabilitation. among the measured signals, biopotential is detected by well-known medical techniques, such as electrocardiography (ECG), electroencephalography (EEG), electromyography (EMG), and electrooculography (EOG) to track the activity of heart, brain, muscles, and eyes, respectively [3, 4]. For instance, EMG signal is exploited to obtain information about muscular activity for diagnosis or rehabilitation purposes, as well as an input to trigger active devices, such as human-machine interfaces and prostheses [5]. State of art EMG devices are usually bulky and require different cables that could be uncomfortable for the final user. To overcome those problems wearable devices are lately arising. These

© ICST Institute for Computer Sciences, Social Informatics and Telecommunications Engineering 2021
Published by Springer Nature Switzerland AG 2021. All Rights Reserved
R. Goleva et al. (Eds.): HealthyIoT 2020, LNICST 360, pp. 55–60, 2021.
https://doi.org/10.1007/978-3-030-69963-5_4

devices have small dimensions and they can be worn and carried by the users without interfering with their everyday life improving both the user experience and the quality of collected data. Wearables EMG devices were lately explored for example to remotely monitor patients [6], evaluate neck fatigue [7] and discriminate wrist gestures [8]. In this work we propose a novel wearable device to perform EMG acquisition using a compact electronic board and a matrix of electrodes fabricated by aerosol jet printing (AJP) that can be used in remote rehabilitation or training applications. This device is able to provide a real-time, reliable, wireless data transmission to provide data to a custom application running on a remote unit that can be both a pc or a mobile phone that can send feedback to a clinician to remotely monitor a patient's improvement during remote rehabilitation. In Sect. 2, we discuss the design process and the system's architecture that is later tested and validated in Sect. 3.

## 2    Materials and Methods

### 2.1    Device Design

The overall system's architecture (Fig. 1) consists of two main parts: a wearable unit and a remote one. The former acquires signals from the human body through the electrodes, converts them to digital ones and sends them through Bluetooth Low Energy (BLE) to the remote unit that is devoted to store the data, perform pre-processing steps and provide the results to custom applications.

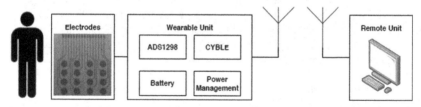

**Fig. 1.** The architecture of the system.

### 2.2    Electrode Fabrication

A matrix of 16 electrodes to achieve an 8 channel EMG was designed and fabricated by aerosol jet printing (AJP). This matrix configuration allows monitoring different parts of a muscle to analyze its functionality and the signal transmission, or to interface EMG signals realizing a human-machine interface. AJP is a fully additive printing method that atomizes an ink and deposes it with a sheath gas through a nozzle. With this technique, it is possible to depose a wide set of inks in a low-temperature environment on substrates that are not conventional for electronics, like plastic sheets and paper. The matrix of 16 electrodes was printed (Fig. 2) using the Novacentrix Metalon HPS-108AE1, silver nanoflakes based ink on a photographic paper. This combination allows to achieve flexibility, low-cost, biocompatibility and sustainability (it can be burned after use) and thus simplifies the adhesion between the electrodes and non-planar surface of the body.

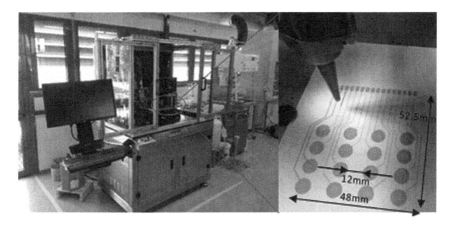

**Fig. 2.** Matrix electrode during the fabrication

## 2.3 Wearable Unit

The 52.5 mm × 48.0 mm electrode matrix is connected with the wearable unit that implements analog signal conditioning, signal sampling, data organization and transmission. In Fig. 3 the device block scheme is depicted. In order to optimize device dimensions, its power requirements and its efficiency, the design mostly uses off-the-shelf integrated circuits (IC) and minimizes the number of required components. ADS1298 by Texas Instruments was selected to provide a dedicated analog front-end (AFE) and a 24-bit delta-sigma $\Delta\Sigma$ analog-to-digital converter (ADC) to each of its 8 differential channels. This device is controlled by Serial Peripheral Interface (SPI) commands and allows different gains (the possible are: 1, 2, 3, 4, 6, 8, or 12) and sampling frequencies. To define this last parameter, we considered that most of EMG signal's information is situated below 500 Hz and thus we decided to use a minimum sampling frequency fs = 1 kHz. As regards the gain, in the experimental setup, we finally defined as reliable a value of 12. All the 8 differential channels are sampled synchronously and when the data is ready they are collected through SPI as a 27-Byte array called sample (it also includes a 3 Byte status word that provides information about the ADS1298 status e.g. the values of its GPIOs) by CYBLE-222014–01 Cypress Semiconductor microcontroller. This component controls the device behavior and integrates also a BLE module to transmit towards the remote unit the EMG data. The BLE module was set using the microcontroller API to be a GATT server and to produce a notification event when a packet is ready. The fabricated printed circuit board (PCB) has a dimension of 4.5 cm × 4.5 cm printed circuit board (PCB). This includes the already described components, several required passive components and a TPS709 Texas Instruments voltage regulator that provides a stable 3.3 V supply voltage. The maximum current absorption of 55 mA was estimated for the device during the elaboration and BLE communication. With these specifications (using fs = 1 kHz, 18 ms are required to collect the data), we estimated an average transmission time of 9.5 ms, thus ensuring a possible real-time communication; the maximum transmission time is 65 ms and thus, to avoid overwriting packets, a circular output buffer was introduced.

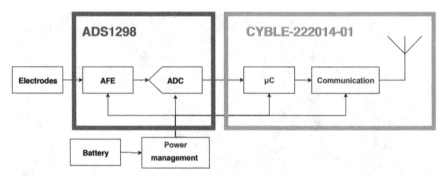

**Fig. 3.** Block scheme of the wearable unit where the main used components are underlined.

## 2.4  Remote Unit

The remote unit performs specific communication tasks with the wearable unit in order to configure it and to retrieve data from it. Moreover, the remote unit elaborates, stores and displays the incoming data. CY5677 - CySmart Bluetooth Low Energy 4.2 USB Dongle by Cypress Semiconductors was selected to interface via BLE the wearable unit and a PC to collect and save data in real-time. A dedicated program to elaborate, visualize and save as.csv files the data. Those files could be used to feed some application programs for example to track signal propagation on muscles, evaluate muscles damages, deduce activation patterns and upload on an online database the collected information.

## 2.5  Testing and Validation

To validate the proposed approach, at first, a signal generator was connected to one of the input channels of the wearable device to verify the correct implementation of the data retrieval and transmission towards the remote unit. In order to optimize the communication with the wearable unit, different packet lengths were tested, and the average and maximum transmission time were measured. Each BLE packet provides different additional information including the incremental number that allowed to track how many packets were received correctly, how long it takes to receive a defined packet and the average throughput. Thanks to this information it is possible to evaluate the overall efficacy of the communication measuring from the remote unit these key parameters. As experimental setup, the wearable device and the remote unit were positioned less than 2 m afar and then we started collecting data for different periods of time from 41.67 s up to 486 s. According to the preliminary experimental results we chose to put in each packet 500 B to store 18 samples and a successive packet identifier.

Furthermore, to validate the proposed wearable device in an application-like fashion, we performed a measure on a healthy volunteer. The printed matrix of 16 electrodes was attached to the brachial biceps using an electroconductive gel to improve the electrodes performances. The electrodes were wired and connected to the PCB. It was required to the subject to follow a pattern mixing maximal isometric contractions with rough duration of 30 s with relaxation periods. The retrieved signals were conditioned and analyzed in both time- and frequency-domain on the remote unit by using MATLAB and including digital notch filters to remove all the 50 Hz harmonics. A proper comparison between commercial and printed electrodes was reported in [9] where is stated that printed electrodes have slightly worse performances than the commercial ones but on the other hand, they present a reduced encumbrance and thickness that are better on the wearability and conformability on the body.

## 3 Results

From the measurements performed during the transmission test, an average throughput of (27 763 ± 19) B/s was calculated considering that more than 99.7% of the packets were delivered correctly. As regards the transmission time, a mean value of (18.01 ± 0.01) ms was measured for the average transmission time ánd (63.4 ± 7.0) ms for the maximum transmission time that confirms the values that we used to design the device.

During the system validation on a healthy subject, we were able to correctly retrieve EMG signal on each channel (Fig. 4), where it is possible to clearly distinguish between contraction and relaxation of the muscles. We also observed different spikes on the signals probably due to wiring movements during the acquisition.

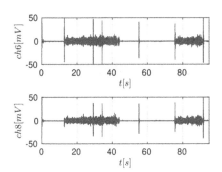

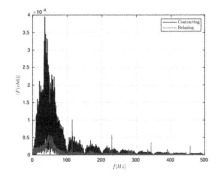

**Fig. 4.** Resulting signals after digital filtering

**Fig. 5.** FFT of the signal on one of the channels. In blue we present the contraction periods and in red the relaxation ones (Color figure online)

Then a fast Fourier transform (FFT) of the signals was performed dividing them between contraction and relaxation of the muscle. Figure 5 shows that most of the energy of the signals during contraction was before 150 Hz as expected. Moreover, we were able to observe both the influence of the filters and noise components introduced by the analog front-end, that are well visible analyzing the relaxed signal. It was also observed the energy difference between the two sets of data. Signal to noise ratio (SNR) was calculated using the RMS value of the contraction (that we used as signal) and the relaxation period (that we used as noise sample). We obtained an SNR of the whole circuit higher than 28 dB. This result can be improved by modifying the electrode geometry such as increasing the area of the electrodes and their adhesion on the muscles.

## 4 Conclusions

In this work, a novel wearable device to perform a multichannel EMG using an AJP printed matrix of electrodes is shown. The proposed solution allows for flexibility, low-cost, biocompatibility, sustainability and less invasiveness. This device provides a real-time stream of data from wearable to remote unit using BLE achieving an average throughput of 27 763 B/s with a success rate sending packets above 99.7%. The device samples eight channels at fs = 1 kHz and this limits the useful signal the bandwidth to 500 Hz. On the remote unit, a set of digital filters were developed to attenuate spurious components and thus improve the SNR to 28 dB. This device exploiting the potentiality of IoT can be used to provide data to a remote unit to perform different tasks as detect activation patterns, monitor muscles fatigue and integrity.

## References

1. Borghetti, M., Serpelloni, M., Sardini, E., Casas, O.: Multisensor system for analyzing the thigh movement during walking. IEEE Sens. J. **15**, 4953–4961 (2017)
2. Mekki, F., Borghetti, M., Sardini, E., Serpelloni, M.: Wireless instrumented cane for walking monitoring in parkinson patients. In: 2017 IEEE International Symposium on Medical Measurements and Applications (MeMeA), pp. 414–419 (2017)
3. Trung, T.Q., Lee, N.E.: Flexible and stretchable physical sensor integrated platforms for wearable human-activity monitoring and personal healthcare. Adv. Mater. **22**, 4338–4372 (2016)
4. Chlaihawi, A.A., Narakathu, B.B., Emamian, S., Bazuin, B.J., Atashbar, M.Z.: Development of printed and flexible dry ECG electrodes. Sens. Bio-Sens. Res. **20**, 9–15 (2018)
5. Kim, N., Lim, T., Song, K., Yang, S., Lee, J.: Stretchable multichannel electromyography sensor array covering large area for controlling home electronics with distinguishable signals from multiple muscles. ACS Appl. Mater. Interfaces **32**, 21070–21076 (2016)
6. Ishak, A.J., Ahmad, S.A., Soh, A.C., Naraina, N.A., Jusoh, R.M.R., Chikamune, W.: Design of a wireless surface EMG acquisition system. IEEE (2017)
7. Choi, H.S.: EMG sensor system for neck fatigue assessment using RF wireless power transmission. IEEE (2018)
8. Higashi, S., Goto, D., Okada, S., Shiozawa, N., Makikawa, M.: Development of wearable EMG measurement system on forearm for wrist gestures discrimination. IEEE (2019)
9. Borghetti, M., Fapanni, T., Lopomo, N.F., Sardini, E., Serpelloni, M.: A preliminary study on aerosol jet-printed stretchable dry electrode for electromyography. In: Saponara, S., De Gloria, A. (eds.) Applications in Electronics Pervading Industry, Environment and Society. ApplePies 2020. Lecture Notes in Electrical Engineering, vol. 738. Springer, Cham (2021). https://doi.org/10.1007/978-3-030-66729-0_36

# Chronic Kidney Disease Early Diagnosis Enhancing by Using Data Mining Classification and Features Selection

Pedro A. Moreno-Sanchez[(⊠)] (iD)

School of Health Care and Social Work, Seinäjoki University of Applied Sciences,
60100 Seinäjoki, Finland
pedro.morenosanchez@seamk.fi

**Abstract.** Chronic Kidney Disease (CKD) is currently a worldwide chronic disease with an increasing incidence, prevalence and high cost to health systems. A delayed recognition and prevention often lead to a premature mortality due to progressive and incurable loss of kidney function. Data mining classifiers employment to discover patterns in CKD indicators would contribute to an early diagnosis that allow patients to prevent such kidney severe damage. Adopting the cross Industry Standard Process of Data Mining (CRISP-DM) methodology, this work develops a classifier model that would support healthcare professionals in early diagnosis of CKD patients. By building a data pipeline that manages the different phases of CRISP-DM, an automated data transformation, modelling and evaluation is applied to the CKD dataset extracted from the UCI ML repository. Moreover, the pipeline along with the Scikit-learn package's GridSearchCV is used to carry out an exhaustive search of the best data mining classifier and the different parameters of the data preparation's sub-stages like data missing and feature selection. Thus, AdaBoost is selected as the best classifier and it outperforms with a 100% in terms of accuracy, precision, sensivity, specificity, f1-score and roc auc, the classification results obtained by the related works reviewed. Moreover, the application of feature selection reduces up to 12 out of 24 features which are employed in the classifier model developed.

**Keywords:** Chronic kidney disease · Early diagnosis · Data mining · Classification · Feature selection

## 1 Introduction

Chronic kidney disease (CKD) is a worldwide public health problem with an increasing incidence, prevalence, and high cost to health systems. Globally, in 2017, 1.2 million people died from CKD, increasing the all-age mortality rate up to 41.5% since 1990. The same year, a number of 697.5 million cases of all-stage CKD were recorded that implies a global prevalence of 9,1% [1]. CKD is the most common type of kidney diseases that lead a vast majority of CKD patients to suffer premature mortality due to cardiovascular

© ICST Institute for Computer Sciences, Social Informatics and Telecommunications Engineering 2021
Published by Springer Nature Switzerland AG 2021. All Rights Reserved

R. Goleva et al. (Eds.): HealthyIoT 2020, LNICST 360, pp. 61–76, 2021.
https://doi.org/10.1007/978-3-030-69963-5_5

disease and the progressive loss of kidney function; as well as other types of kidney-injured syndromes with significant negative effects on their quality of life and survival rate [2].

Typically, CKD presents no symptoms in an early stage, but later, symptoms may appear like leg swelling, extreme fatigue and generalized weakness, shortness of breath, loss of appetite, or confusion. Slowing the progression of the kidney damage, usually by controlling the underlying causes, is the main focus of CKD treatment. A delayed recognition and prevention often lead to further kidney injury and health problems where hemodialysis or even kidney transplantation are the only way to keep the patient alive [3, 4]. However, the diagnosis of CKD is a process of 3 months where the level Glomerular Filtration Rate (GFR) is assessed, although is not practical for daily clinical use due to complexity of the measure procedure [5, 6]. Therefore, other estimation approaches of GFR, like Cockcroft-Gault equation or Modification of Diet in Renal Disease equation [7], are widely accepted by using filtration markers or risk factors which are easily collected like hypertension, obesity, heart disease, age, diabetes, drug abuse, family history of kidney disease, race/ethnicity [8]. By having the disease diagnosed at the beginning phase the corresponding treatments can be initiated and the patient can live longer even with these insufficient kidney functions.

However, an opaque relationship between CKD and various symptoms exists, thus, data mining is appropriate to discover the latent correlation between them contributing significantly to assess individuals with potential CKD risk. Data mining provides useful tools for multivariate data analysis, namely classification and regression, allowing predictions based on the established models and hence offering a suitable advantage for risk assessment of many diseases including CKD [9]. Therefore, as early detection and proper treatments are the cornerstone to prevent CKD, automated and accurate diagnosis methods of CKD based on data mining are necessary to assist medical personnel to early discover patients at risk and so increase their quality of life expectation.

Large amounts of complex data are being generated by healthcare stakeholders about patients, diseases, hospitals, medical equipment, claims, treatment cost, etc. that requires processing and analysis for knowledge extraction [10]. Machine learning and data mining had been successfully applied, over the past few decades, to build computer-aided diagnosis (CAD) systems for diagnosing complex health issues with good accuracy and efficiency by recognizing potentially useful, original, and comprehensible patterns in health data [11, 12]. Data Mining is particularly useful in medicine when no availability of evidence favoring a certain treatment option is found. Classification is a data mining technique, which belongs to supervised learning methods, with the primary objective of forecasting target classes precisely and accurately for a given case.

This paper aims at enhancing the quality of CKD early diagnosis by developing an automated and accurate classifier model of CKD patients based on data preprocessing and feature selection techniques, as well as an exhaustive search of the best data mining classifier. The main contributions achieved are: a data management pipeline that provides an automated control of classification task and its previous data preparation; a classifier model that outperforms the related works reviewed not only in the training but also in testing phase with new unseen data; and a reduced group of features from the original dataset which are employed by the model to obtain high accurate results in classifying CKD patients.

The next sections of the paper are organized as follows: Sect. 2 shows related works in the CKD diagnosis field, Sect. 3 discusses the methodology employed to build the classifier model, Sect. 4 and 5 shows and discusses the results obtained respectively, and Sect. 6 points the conclusions drawn in this research.

## 2 Related Works

Several data mining approaches have been considered for the detection of CKDs in the literature dealing with either medical images or clinical indicators. In these works, different classifiers have been mainly used such as Logistic Regression (LR), K-Nearest Neighbors (KNN), Support Vector Machines (SVM), Decision Trees (DT), Näive Bayes (NB), Random Forest (RF), Ensemble Learning (Adaboost, Bagging, etc.), and Artificial Neural Networks (ANN).

Despite good accurate results achieved in detecting CKD through data mining classifiers by Chiu et al. (94,75% accuracy) [13], Baby et al. (100% accuracy) [14], or Lakshim et al. (93.85% accuracy) [15]; a comparison cannot be carried out due to different datasets employed in the classification task. However, other different studies that employed, like this research, the CKD dataset from UCI repository [16] are described as following with the aim at comparing them to our results.

Different classifiers as Radial Basis Function (RBF), LR and Multilayer perceptron (MLP) were assessed by Rubini et al. [17] being the MLP the best one with results as: 99.75% accuracy, 99.66% F1-score, 99.33% recall and 100% specificity. Ani et al. [18] built a clinical decision support system for CKD risk prediction comparing several classifier and ranking its accuracy: BackProp neural network (81.5%), NB (78%), LDA (76%), KNN(90%), DT (93%), and Random subspace classification algorithms (94%). Other classifiers (KNN, SVM, LR, DT) were explored by Charleonnan et al. [19], being SVM the most accurate (98,3%) with a sensivity of 99% and specificity of 98%. Chen et al. [2] also demonstrated SVM had better accuracy (99.7%) over other methods as KNN or soft independent modeling of class analogy (SIMCA) in classifying CKD. In their research, Kunwar et al. [10] showed that NB outperforms ANN in accuracy (100% over 72.73%). Jeewantha et al. applied the percentage split method on the dataset, demonstrating most classifiers have better accuracy when percentage of training data is higher, with the MLP as the most accurate model (98.66%). The only study identified where cross-validation technique were not applied was performed by Imran et al. [11] obtaining a 99% of F1-score, precision, recall and area under the curve ROC (Roc Auc) with a model based on Feedforward neural networks over unseen samples of the test set. In addition, Van Eyck et al. [20] achieved in 2016 the best results so far with a 100% in terms of accuracy, precision, sensivity and specificity by using RF.

On the other hand, other studies explored the influence of feature selection in the classifiers result. Thus, Chetty et al. [21] applied different classifiers along with wrapper feature selection methods demonstrating that the classifiers tested performed better on reduced dataset than the original with an accuracy of 100% by using best first search strategy in wrapper feature selection and KNN classifier. Salekin et al. [7] found RF had better accuracy (99%) than KNN and ANN when wrapper feature selection or Lasso with 12 or 10 features respectively was applied. The combination of RF with feature selection as the most accurate (99.75%) was confirmed by Siyad et al. [22] among other as NB (97.5%), LR (98%) or DT(98%). Feature selection was also tested by Basar et al. [23] on ensemble classifiers like AdaBoost, Bagging or Random Subspaces, being the latter the best one with 100% of accuracy by considering only 10 features of the original UCI dataset. Wibawa et al. [24] added another research to works on testing ensemble classifiers with feature selection, having an accuracy of 98,1% and 98% as F-score, prediction and recall in a resultant dataset of 17 features with AdaBoost-KNN classifiers. In the same line, Zubair et al. [25] obtained an accuracy of 99% by using AdaBoost classifier plus ExtraTree to select the 13 most important features.

**Table 1.** Classification results (expressed in %) of related works. *: *cross-validation technique not applied*

| Article | Accuracy | F1-Score | Precision | Specificity | Recall | Roc Auc |
|---|---|---|---|---|---|---|
| *Rubini* [17] | 100 | 100 | – | 100 | 99 | – |
| *Basar* [23] | 100 | – | – | – | – | – |
| *Van Eyck* [20] | 100 | – | 100 | 100 | 100 | 100 |
| *Ani* [18] | 94 | 95 | 97 | – | 93 | – |
| *Chen* [2] | 100 | – | – | – | 100 | – |
| *Chetty* [21] | 100 | – | – | – | – | – |
| *Kunwar* [10] | 100 | – | – | – | – | – |
| *Jeewantha* [8] | 99 | – | – | – | – | 100 |
| *Salekin* [7] | – | 99 | – | – | – | – |
| *Wibawa* [24] | 98 | 98 | 98 | – | 98 | – |
| *Zubair* [25] | 99 | 99 | – | – | – | – |
| *Charleonnan* [19] | 98 | – | – | 98 | 99 | – |
| *Siyad* [22] | 100 | – | – | – | – | – |
| *Imran* [11](*) | 99 | 97 | – | – | 99 | 99 |

As Table 1 shows, the results obtained by the different studies are almost perfect in terms of accuracy (values close to 100%). However, it must be noted that all papers reviewed, except one (Imran et al. [11]), performed the cross-validation technique to obtain their results. This technique allows using every sample of the dataset to train the model. Only Imran's model was performed over unseen data samples. Therefore, the rest of models' performance would be unknown in a deployment phase with data that have not been used for training.

# 3   Material and Methods

For this study, the Cross-Industry Standard Process for Data Mining (CRISP-DM) has been adopted [26]. CRISP-DM gives a methodological way to manage data mining development. As shown in Fig. 1, CRISP-DM establishes a continuous loop composed of 6 steps: Business Understanding, Data Understanding, Data Preparation, Modeling, Evaluation, Deployment.

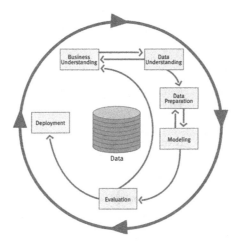

**Fig. 1.** CRISP-DM methodology [26].

With the aim at improving the automation and efficiency in building the classifier model as well as deploying it in a real-world scenario, developers usually combine the phases of data preparation, modelling and evaluation into a data management pipeline that controls the data flow through all algorithms applied.

## 3.1   Business Understanding

This stage is the most important because the intention of the project is outlined here. The main objective of this research work is to achieve a data mining model that guarantees a highly accurate and efficient classification of CKD patients.

## 3.2   Data Understanding

This step begins with an underlying data gathering and continues with actions to facilitate the understanding of what the project wants and needs in terms of data.

As mentioned before, the CKD dataset used in this research was extracted from the UCI Machine Learning Repository [16]. The data set, collected from the Apollo Hospitals, Karaikudi, India during a nearly 2-month period in 2015, includes a total of 400 samples depicted by 11 numeric, 13 nominal attributes and a class attribute (ckd/notckd). Out of 400 samples, 250 samples belonged to the CKD group (62.5%), and the other 150 samples to the non-CKD group implying an imbalanced dataset. Table 2 lists the attributes from the original data set. It must be noted every attribute contained missing values except the class attribute, due to possibly to the fault of the receiver input, sensor error or reluctance on data resource. The indicators considered in this dataset are feasible to collect [7] in clinical routine favoring an early diagnosis of CKD.

**Table 2.** Attributes description of CKD dataset

|    | Attributes [Acronym] | Indication | Average/nominal values |
|----|----------------------|------------|------------------------|
| 1  | Age (year) [age] | Numerical | 51.5 (avg) |
| 2  | Blood pressure (mm/Hg) [bp] | Numerical | 76.5 (avg) |
| 3  | Specific gravity [sg] | Nominal (1.005, 1.010, 1.015, 1.020, 1.025) | 7, 84, 75, 106, 81 |
| 4  | Albumin [al] | Nominal (0, 1, 2, 3, 4, 5) | 199, 44, 43, 43, 24, 1 |
| 5  | Sugar [su] | Nominal (0, 1, 2, 3, 4, 5) | 290, 13, 18, 14, 13, 3 |
| 6  | Red blood cells [rbc] | Normal or abnormal | 47 abnormal |
| 7  | Pus cell [pc] | Normal or abnormal | 76 abnormal |
| 8  | Pus cell clumps [pcc] | Present or not present | 42 present |
| 9  | Bacteria [ba] | Present or not present | 22 present |
| 10 | Blood glucose random (mgs/dl) [bgr] | Numerical | 148.04 (avg) |
| 11 | Blood urea (mgs/dl) [bu] | Numerical | 57.43 (avg) |
| 12 | Serum creatinine (mgs/dl) [sc] | Numerical | 3.07 (avg) |
| 13 | Sodium (mEq/l) [sod] | Numerical | 137.53 (avg) |
| 14 | Potassium (mEq/l) [pot] | Numerical | 4.63 (avg) |
| 15 | Hemoglobin (gms) [hemo] | Numerical | 12.53 (avg) |
| 16 | Packed cell volume [pcv] | Numerical | 38.88 (avg) |
| 17 | White blood cell count (cells/cumm) [wc] | Numerical | 8406.12 (avg) |
| 18 | Red blood cell count (cells/cumm) [rc] | Numerical | 4.71 (avg) |
| 19 | Hypertension [htn] | Yes or no | 147 yes |
| 20 | Diabetes mellitus [dm] | Yes or no | 137 yes |
| 21 | Coronary artery disease [cad] | Yes or no | 34 yes |
| 22 | Appetite [appet] | Good or poor | 82 poor |
| 23 | Pedal edema [pe] | Yes or no | 76 yes |
| 24 | Anemia [ane] | Yes or no | 60 yes |
| 25 | Target class | ckd or notckd | 250 ckd |

### 3.3 Data Preparation

Once the data has been collected, it must be transformed or preprocessed into a usable subset by checking for questionable, missing or ambiguous cases.

Missing value imputation is one of the important tasks in data mining especially in the cases where the data is small and there is a need of using all available data, as occurs with CKD dataset [9]. For handling data missing values several approaches can be followed depending on the type of attribute or feature. Regarding numerical features, replacement can be done by Bayesian imputation with median or mean of the rest of feature's values; or applying multivariate imputation through techniques as KNN or iterative correlation among all features. In case of nominal features, the most common approach is to substitute missing value for the most common value of the feature.

Relatively many features can overload the classifier contributing negatively towards the calculation of the classification as well as increasing the computational time. Feature subset selection aims to reduce computing time and improve the results of prediction by removing the features/attributes in a dataset that are considered unimportant or unable to contribute to accuracy of the classification [17]. Features selection method also depends on the input feature category and the target class' category, although there are methods that can be used for both like mutual information or recursive feature elimination (RFE). Apart from the two latter, this study will use ANOVA and Chi-Squared (Chi$^2$) for numerical and nominal categories respectively.

Another technique used in data preparation is feature scaling to allow the model to process the samples of numerical features with a normalized range of values by applying for instance minmax scaling (used here) or standard scaling. On the other hand, nominal features are usually encoded into numbers to allow the model to perform correctly.

### 3.4 Modeling

Once data is prepared for being processed, several data mining classifiers can be applied in order to discover underlying patterns and so to gain meaningful insights. This is the purpose of data mining: to create knowledge information that has meaning and utility.

Depending on the data mining tasks, models used can be classifiers or regressors. As the goal of this research was to enhance early diagnosis of CKD patients through classification, the following classifiers employed were: Logistic Regression, Support Vector Machine, Decision Trees, Random Forest, Multilayer Perceptron, Naïve Bayes, K-Nearest Neighbors, and AdaBoost with Decision Tree as base classifier. These classifiers have been employed in related works described previously, and their usage will allow to compare the performance of the model developed in this research.

### 3.5 Evaluation

Classifier model selection must be done by dealing with a portion of the data and adjustments are made if necessary. Therefore, splitting the training set is recommended in this phase to divide in into a training subset, to decide which model performs better, and a validation subset, to tweak the hyperparameters of the selected model refining the classification accuracy. The k-fold cross-validation technique allows using each sample of the dataset for training k-1 times and testing 1 time [27]. Therefore, the variance of classification result can be minimized. However, the dataset should have been previously split to save a test set with the aim to run the model on unseen data, thus, ensuring new samples will be classified as expected in the next deployment phase. In this research, a test set is firstly generated, and the cross-validation technique is used on training set to select the model and the parameters of the data preparation phase.

To estimate classification performance, several metrics are used in this research, namely: accuracy, precision, recall/sensitivity, specificity, f1-score and roc-auc. Accuracy describes the rate of true predictions and it is suitable for balanced data among classes. However, because the data on CKD dataset is not balanced, the other metrics will be used to assess the model classifier. As following, the formulas of the measures used are shown considering the acronyms depicted in the confusion matrix (Tables 3 and 4).

**Table 3.** Confusion matrix layout

|  |  | Predicted class | |
|---|---|---|---|
|  |  | 0 | 1 |
| Actual class | 0 | TN (True Negative) | FP (False Positive) |
|  | 1 | FN (False Negative) | TP (True Positive) |

**Table 4.** Classification metrics formula

| Classification metrics | Formula |
|---|---|
| *Accuracy*: the overall success rate of true prediction | $\frac{(TP+TN)}{(TP+TN+FP+FN)}$ (1) |
| *Sensitivity/Recall*: fraction of positive instances predicted correctly | $\frac{TP}{(TP+FN)}$ (2) |
| *Specificity*: fraction of negative instances predicted correctly | $\frac{TN}{(FP+TN)}$ (3) |
| *Precision:* fraction of true positive data given all true predicted data | $\frac{TP}{(TP+FP)}$ (4) |
| *F1-Score*: harmonic mean from precision and recall | $2 * (\frac{Precision*Recall}{Precision+Recall})$ (5) |

*Roc-Auc*: Area under curve ROC (Receiver Operating Characteristic). Values between 0 and 1 and higher values imply better classification performance

### 3.6 Deployment

This stage is envisioned to put the selected model to perform on new data in a production environment in line with the project's objectives. Concerning this research, in this phase the model selected would be performed in clinical routine. The new interactions at this phase might reveal the new variables and needs for the dataset and model. These new challenges could initiate revision of either business needs and actions, or the model and data, or both.

## 3.7  Data Mining Software

In this research, Python [28] has been used as language programming along with scikit-learn package [29] that allows to develop every stage of the CRISP-DM methodology. In particular, by using the scikit-learn's module GridSearchCV, multiple combinations of classifiers, data missing imputation, scaling and feature selection techniques have been tested to find the best model to classify CKD.

# 4  Results

## 4.1  CKD Classifier Experimental Setup

As mentioned before, developers are encouraged to build pipelines that manage the data operations tackled in the data preparation, modelling and evaluation phases of CRISP-DM methodology.

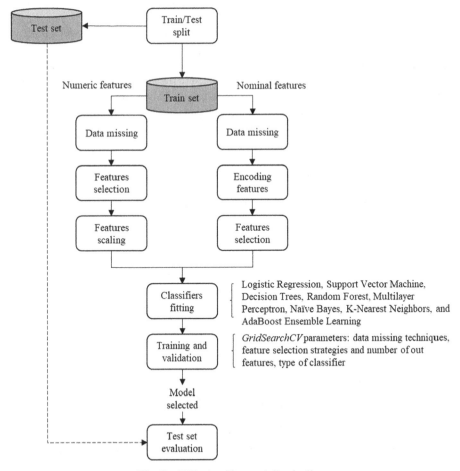

**Fig. 2.** CKD classifier model's pipeline

Figure 2 shows the different steps of the data management pipeline developed in this research that allows to find the best model to classify CKD patients. As a previous step, the original dataset was split for training (70% i.e. 280 samples) and testing (30% i.e. 120 samples), maintaining the same proportion of ckd/non-ckd in both sets. Next, the first step of this two-branch pipeline entails the separation of numerical and nominal features. Regarding numeric features, data missing techniques are applied first and then continuing with selection of those relevant features and a further scaling applying mixmax normalization. Data missing is also tackled first in nominal features and before applying feature selection, these features are encoded into numbers to ensure a correct performance in further steps. In order to select the model which performs the best classification of CKD patients, the classifier is trained and then validated by using 5-fold cross-validation. For that purpose, the scikit-learn's module GridSearchCV was employed since it allows to find the best classifier applying cross-validation as well as trying a grid of parameters for every stage of the pipeline. Finally, samples from the test set were used with the best model found to evaluate its classification performance with unseen data. This last evaluation gives a real notion about the selected model's performance with new data (i.e. data not used for training).

GridSearchCV allows developers to find the best combination of a model's parameters by applying an exhaustive search with multiple candidates generated from a pre-defined grid of parameters. Therefore, in this research the parameters needed to be optimized for the best resultant model corresponded to data missing techniques, feature selection strategy and its number of output features, as well as the type of data mining classifier employed. Table 5 shows the different values considered for these parameters.

**Table 5.** GridSearch CV parameters employed

| GridSearchCV parameters | Values |
|---|---|
| Data missing strategy for numeric features | Mean, median, KNN, iterative |
| Feature selection strategy | ANOVA (only numeric features), $Chi^2$ (only nominal features), mutual information, Recursive Feature Elimination (RFE) |
| Number of output features | 1 to 11 for numeric; 1 to 13 for nominal |
| Classifiers | Logistic Regression, Support Vector Machine, Decision Trees, Random Forest, Multilayer Perceptron, Naïve Bayes, K-Nearest Neighbors, and AdaBoost with decision tree as base classifier |

## 4.2   CKD Classification and Feature Selection Results

According to GridSearchCV results, the best model's parameters found were: median for data missing strategy; RFE and 4 output features for numeric features; RFE and 5 output features for nominal features; and AdaBoost classifier. The first 3 best combination found by GridSearchCV results are shown in Table 6.

**Table 6.** Best 3 models found by GridSearchCV (all cells expressed in %)

| Best Model (classifier, data missing, numeric feature selection, nominal feature selection) | Accuracy | F1-Score | Precision | Specificity | Recall | Roc Auc |
|---|---|---|---|---|---|---|
| AdaBoost, median, RFE#4, RFE#5 | 100 | 100 | 100 | 100 | 100 | 100 |
| AdaBoost, median, ANOVA#7; Chi$^2$#7 | 99.64 | 99.53 | 99.09 | 99.42 | 100 | 99.71 |
| AdaBoost, median, ANOVA#7, RFE#5 | 99.64 | 99.51 | 100 | 100 | 99.04 | 99.52 |

Moreover, Table 7 shows a comparison of the cross-validation results using the different classifiers but maintaining the best model's parameters related to data missing and feature selection.

**Table 7.** Comparison of best model parameters with all classifier considered (all cells expressed in %)

| Classifier | Accuracy | F1-Score | Precision | Specificity | Recall | Roc Auc |
|---|---|---|---|---|---|---|
| AdaBoost | 100 | 100 | 100 | 100 | 100 | 100 |
| Random Forest | 99.29 | 99.00 | 100 | 100 | 98.10 | 99.05 |
| Multilayer Perceptron | 98.57 | 98.16 | 96.44 | 97.71 | 100 | 98.86 |
| Logistic Regression | 98.21 | 97.70 | 95.53 | 97.14 | 100 | 98.57 |
| Decision Trees | 98.21 | 97.67 | 97.50 | 98.29 | 98.10 | 98.19 |
| Support Vector Machine | 97.86 | 97.29 | 94.85 | 96.57 | 100 | 98.29 |
| K-Nearest Neighbors | 97.86 | 97.29 | 94.85 | 96.57 | 100 | 98.29 |
| Naïve Bayes | 95.71 | 94.61 | 89.78 | 93.14 | 100 | 96.57 |

The final step of the pipeline proposed in this research entailed the evaluation of the best model achieved on the test set's samples to see its performance with new unseen data. The 3 best models extracted in GridSearchCV results were evaluated in these conditions and classification results are shown in Table 8:

**Table 8.** 3 best models found by GridSearchCV evaluated on test set (all cells expressed in %)

| Best model | Accuracy | F1-Score | Precision | Specificity | Recall | Roc Auc |
|---|---|---|---|---|---|---|
| AdaBoost, median, RFE#4, RFE#5 | 98.33 | 98.34 | 98.40 | 98.33 | 98.83 | 98.67 |
| AdaBoost, median, ANOVA#7; Chi$^2$#7 | 99.17 | 99.17 | 99.18 | 99.17 | 99.17 | 99.33 |
| AdaBoost, median, ANOVA#7, RFE#5 | 100 | 100 | 100 | 100 | 100 | 100 |

The confusion matrix of these models by using the samples of test set (120 samples) are depicted in Table 9.

**Table 9.** Confusion matrix of best selected models with samples of test set.

| | | | Predicted class | |
|---|---|---|---|---|
| | | | ckd | notckd |
| AdaBoost, median, RFE#4, RFE#5 | **Actual class** | ckd | 73 | 2 |
| | | notckd | 0 | 45 |
| AdaBoost, median, ANOVA#7; Chi$^2$#7 | **Actual class** | ckd | 74 | 1 |
| | | notckd | 0 | 45 |
| AdaBoost, median, ANOVA#7, RFE#5 | **Actual class** | ckd | 75 | 0 |
| | | notckd | 0 | 45 |

In addition, the best models indicated that only 9, 12 and 14 out of 24 features were considered as relevant to achieve such results. The features selected for the 3 best models are shown in Table 10.

**Table 10.** Features selected in the 3 best models found by GridSearchCV

| Best models | Numeric features | Nominal features |
|---|---|---|
| AdaBoost, median, RFE#4, RFE#5 | Serum creatinine, Potassium, Hemoglobin, Red blood cell count | Specific gravity, Albumin, Hypertension, Diabetes mellitus, Pedal edema |
| AdaBoost, median, ANOVA#7; Chi$^2$#7 | Blood glucose random, Blood urea, Serum creatinine, Sodium, Hemoglobin, Packed cell volume, Red blood cell count | Specific gravity, Albumin, Sugar, Hypertension, Diabetes mellitus, Appetite, Pedal edema |
| AdaBoost, median, ANOVA#7, RFE#5 | Blood glucose random, Blood urea, Serum creatinine, Sodium, Hemoglobin, Packed cell volume, Red blood cell count | Specific gravity, Albumin, Hypertension, Diabetes mellitus, Pedal edema |

## 5   Discussion

The pipeline developed in this research offers the possibility to automate not only the training and testing of the model but also the searching of best parameters involved in the data preparation phase as well as the data mining classifier employed. Furthermore, this pipeline would manage classification of new samples in case it appeared, as well as the consequent model retraining and adaptation to new incoming data.

The classification results achieved by this research after applying cross-validation technique through GridSearchCV manifested that the classifier AdaBoost performed a better classification task compared to other classifiers considered. Moreover, such classifier along with the parameters selected by GridSearchCV (median, RFE#4, RFE#5) obtained results of 100% in terms of accuracy, precision, sensivity, specificity, f1-score and Roc Auc. Compared to the results from other related works, this research reached the most accurate figures so far like research developed by Van Eyck et al. [20].

However, the best model selected with cross-validation did not perform as the best with the new data belonging to the test set. Here, a clear example of overfitting existed since the best trained model was not the most accurate in classifying new unseen data. Consequently, other model that involved a bigger number of selected features (ANOVA#7, RFE#5) was evaluated and it classified better since the new information of features added allowed to achieve results of 100% in every classification metric considered. For the best of our knowledge, this research outperforms the rest of studies developed in CKD patients classification so far, because not only equalizing the best model obtained by using cross validation, but also achieving a perfect classification with unseen data which has not been found in any related work. The split of the dataset into a training/validation subset, on one side, and test subset on the other, with a ratio of 70/30 could negatively affect the model performance since a small group of samples were dedicated for training. However, the classification results demonstrated the decision made about developing the pipeline and using the cross-validation strategy developed was correct.

Moreover this study contributes to the state-of-art by proposing a reduced group among the entire dataset's features with several implications: higher feasibility in classifying CKD patients since the number of features to be collected are lower; and a decreasing cost to healthcare systems as extracting less clinical indicators proposed by such features selected.

Due to the fact that the classifier selected is AdaBoost with Decision Tree as base classifier, an exploration of features importance in the classification task could be carried out with the aim at giving healthcare professionals an easier understanding and interpretability of the outcomes generated by the model. By doing so, not only would clinicians achieve an early diagnosis with a reduced group of indicators but also, they could focus on treatment for those important features to the risk of suffering CKD or even revert the disease progress returning to an earlier CKD stage.

## 6   Conclusion

This article shows a development of a classifier model aimed at early diagnosis of Chronic Kidney Disease (CKD) patients. CKD is a worldwide chronic disease with an increasing incidence that leads patients to a premature mortality if it is detected in later stages. A review of the related works has been carried out by depicting the classification results achieved by different authors. The CRISP-DM methodology has been adopted in the classifier model development to ensure data is properly processed. Moreover, a data management pipeline has been developed for automating all stages of data preparation, modeling and evaluation. After applying cross-validation technique through scikit-learn package's GridSearchCV, the best model comprises AdaBoost, as best classifier; and median, RFE#4, RFE#5 as best data preparation's parameters. Next, this best model is also tested with new unseen data by using the test set that has been previously split from the original dataset before using the pipeline developed. Moreover, an exploration of the features selected during the data preparation phase are carried out to depict those dataset's attributes that contribute to the model performance. A case of overfitting is identified since the best trained model performs worse than the other model with more features selected when dealing with unseen data in the testing phase. To the best of our knowledge, the classification results obtained either in cross-validation or in testing phase outperforms the existing results of the related works reviewed.

# References

1. Bikbov, B., et al.: Global, regional, and national burden of chronic kidney disease, 1990–2017: a systematic analysis for the Global Burden of Disease Study 2017. Lancet **395**(10225), 709–733 (2020). https://doi.org/10.1016/S0140-6736(20)30045-3
2. Chen, Z., Zhang, X., Zhang, Z.: Clinical risk assessment of patients with chronic kidney disease by using clinical data and multivariate models. Int. Urol. Nephrol. **48**(12), 2069–2075 (2016). https://doi.org/10.1007/s11255-016-1346-4
3. Keith, D.S., Nichols, G.A., Gullion, C.M., Brown, J.B., Smith, D.H.: Longitudinal follow-up and outcomes among a population with chronic kidney disease in a large managed care organization. Arch. Intern. Med. **164**(6), 659–663 (2004). https://doi.org/10.1001/archinte. 164.6.659
4. Levin, A., et al.: Prevalence of abnormal serum vitamin D, PTH, calcium, and phosphorus in patients with chronic kidney disease: results of the study to evaluate early kidney disease. Kidney Int. **71**(1), 31–38 (2007). https://doi.org/10.1038/sj.ki.5002009
5. Liao, M.-T., Sung, C.-C., Hung, K.-C., Wu, C.-C., Lo, L., Lu, K.-C.: Insulin resistance in patients with chronic kidney disease. J. Biomed. Biotechnol. **2012**, 1–12 (2012). https://www. hindawi.com/journals/bmri/2012/691369/. Accessed 05 Aug 2020
6. Perazella, M.A., Reilly, R.F.: Chronic kidney disease: a new classification and staging system. Hosp. Phys. **39**(3), 18–22 (2003)
7. Salekin, A., Stankovic, J.: Detection of chronic kidney disease and selecting important predictive attributes. In: 2016 IEEE International Conference on Healthcare Informatics (ICHI), pp. 262–270, October 2016. https://doi.org/10.1109/ICHI.2016.36
8. Jeewantha, R.A., Halgamuge, M.N., Mohammad, A., Ekici, G.: Classification performance analysis in medical science: using kidney disease data. In: Proceedings of the 2017 International Conference on Big Data Research, Osaka, Japan, pp. 1–6, October 2017. https://doi. org/10.1145/3152723.3152724
9. Kumar, K., Abhishek, B.: Artificial Neural Networks for Diagnosis of Kidney Stones Disease. GRIN Verlag, Germany (2012)

10. Kunwar, V., Chandel, K., Sabitha, A.S., Bansal, A.: Chronic kidney disease analysis using data mining classification techniques. In: 2016 6th International Conference - Cloud System and Big Data Engineering (Confluence), pp. 300–305, January 2016. https://doi.org/10.1109/CONFLUENCE.2016.7508132

11. Imran, A.A., Amin, M.N., Johora, F.T.: Classification of chronic kidney disease using logistic regression, feedforward neural network and wide deep learning. In: 2018 International Conference on Innovation in Engineering and Technology (ICIET), pp. 1–6, December 2018. https://doi.org/10.1109/CIET.2018.8660844

12. Dhamodharan, S.: Liver disease prediction using Bayesian classification. Int. J. Sci. Eng. Technol. Res. **4**, 3 (2014)

13. Chiu, R.K., Chen, R.Y., Wang, S.-A., Jian, S.-J.: Intelligent systems on the cloud for the early detection of chronic kidney disease. In: 2012 International Conference on Machine Learning and Cybernetics, vol. 5, pp. 1737–1742, July 2012. https://doi.org/10.1109/ICMLC.2012.6359637

14. Baby, P.S., Vital, T.P.: Statistical analysis and predicting kidney diseases using machine learning algorithms. Int. J. Eng. Res. Technol. **4**(7), 206–210 (2015)

15. Lakshmi, K., Nagesh, Y., Krishna, M.V.: Performance comparison of three data mining techniques for predicting kidney dialysis survivability. Int. J. Adv. Eng. Technol. **7**(1), 242 (2014)

16. Dua, D., Graff, C.: UCI Machine Learning Repository. University of California, Irvine, School of Information and Computer Sciences (2017)

17. Rubini, L.J., Eswaran, P.: Generating comparative analysis of early stage prediction of Chronic Kidney Disease. Int. J. Mod. Eng. Res. (IJMER) **5**(7), 49–55 (2015)

18. Ani, R., Sasi, G., Sankar, U.R., Deepa, O.S.: Decision support system for diagnosis and prediction of chronic renal failure using random subspace classification. In: 2016 International Conference on Advances in Computing, Communications and Informatics (ICACCI), pp. 1287–1292, September 2016. https://doi.org/10.1109/ICACCI.2016.7732224

19. Charleonnan, A., Fufaung, T., Niyomwong, T., Chokchueypattanakit, W., Suwannawach, S., Ninchawee, N.: Predictive analytics for chronic kidney disease using machine learning techniques. In: 2016 Management and Innovation Technology International Conference (MITicon), pp. MIT-80–MIT-83, October 2016. https://doi.org/10.1109/MITICON.2016.8025242.

20. Eyck, J.V., et al.: Prediction of chronic kidney disease using random forest machine learning algorithm (2016). https://www.paper/Prediction-of-Chronic-Kidney-Disease-Using-Random-Eyck-Zadeh/c8f5ed96b924f00c729a1a3ff79ead91a8418dc7. Accessed 30 July 2020

21. Chetty, N., Vaisla, K.S., Sudarsan, S.D.: Role of attributes selection in classification of chronic kidney disease patients. In: 2015 International Conference on Computing, Communication and Security (ICCCS), pp. 1–6, December 2015. https://doi.org/10.1109/CCCS.2015.7374193

22. MohammedSiyad, B., Manoj, M.: Fused features classification for the effective prediction of chronic kidney disease. Int. J. **2**, 44–48 (2016)

23. Basar, M.D., Akan, A.: Detection of chronic kidney disease by using ensemble classifiers. In: 2017 10th International Conference on Electrical and Electronics Engineering (ELECO), pp. 544–547, November 2017

24. Wibawa, M.S., Maysanjaya, I.M.D., Putra, I.M.A.W.: Boosted classifier and features selection for enhancing chronic kidney disease diagnose. In: 2017 5th International Conference on Cyber and IT Service Management (CITSM), pp. 1–6, August 2017. https://doi.org/10.1109/CITSM.2017.8089245

25. Zubair Hasan, K.M., Zahid Hasan, M.: Performance evaluation of ensemble-based machine learning techniques for prediction of chronic kidney disease. In: Shetty, N.R., Patnaik, L.M., Nagaraj, H.C., Hamsavath, P.N., Nalini, N. (eds.) Emerging Research in Computing, Information, Communication and Applications. AISC, vol. 882, pp. 415–426. Springer, Singapore (2019). https://doi.org/10.1007/978-981-13-5953-8_34
26. Wirth, R., Hipp, J.: CRISP-DM: towards a standard process model for data mining, p. 11 (2000)
27. Fushiki, T.: Estimation of prediction error by using K-fold cross-validation. Stat. Comput. **21**(2), 137–146 (2011). https://doi.org/10.1007/s11222-009-9153-8
28. Oliphant, T.E.: Python for scientific computing. Comput. Sci. Eng. **9**(3), 10–20 (2007). https://doi.org/10.1109/MCSE.2007.58
29. Pedregosa, F., et al.: Scikit-learn: machine learning in Python. J. Mach. Learn. Res. **12**, 2825–2830 (2011)

# Interpreting the Visual Acuity of the Human Eye with Wearable EEG Device and SSVEP

Danson Evan Garcia[1,2(✉)] ⓘ, Yi Liu[1,2], Kai Wen Zheng[1,2],
Yi (Summer) Tao[1,2], Phillip V. Do[1,2], Cayden Pierce[2], and Steve Mann[1,2]

[1] University of Toronto, Toronto, ON M5S 1A1, Canada
danson.garcia@mail.utoronto.ca
[2] MannLab Canada, Toronto, ON M5T 1G5, Canada

**Abstract.** Using a wearable electroencephalogram (EEG) device, this paper introduces a novel method of quantifying and understanding the visual acuity of the human eye with the steady-state visually evoked potential (SSVEP) technique. This method gives users easy access to self-track and to monitor their eye health. The study focuses on how varying the SSVEP stimulus frequency and duration affect the overall representation of a person's visual perception. The study proposes two methods for this visual representation. The first method is a hardware system that utilizes long-exposure photography to augment reality and collocate the visual map onto the plane of interest. The second is a software implementation that captures the visual field at a set distance. A three-dimensional mapping is created by gathering software-defined visual maps at various set distances. Preliminary results show that these methods can gain some insight into the user's central vision, peripheral vision, and depth perception.

**Keywords:** Wearable sensing · Human monitoring · Electroencephalography · Steady-state visually evoked potentials · Quantified self · Augmented reality

## 1 Background and Introduction

Wearable technology has enabled the "quantified self" movement to transform from a cultural phenomenon into an essential lifestyle [15,36]. The ability to self-track and log various aspects of one's life leads to cheaper and more accessible means of personalized health and wellness care [1,14]. Personal informatics allows users to understand how their body reacts and performs under different scenarios and lifestyles [8]. In effect, wearable technology can act as an early diagnostic tool for detecting undesirable changes to a user's daily functioning.

Wearable electroencephalogram (EEG) devices are an example of wearable technology that tracks user's sleep patterns, mental states, and cognitive health [5]. The collected EEG data can provide immediate feedback to the user

© ICST Institute for Computer Sciences, Social Informatics and Telecommunications Engineering 2021
Published by Springer Nature Switzerland AG 2021. All Rights Reserved
R. Goleva et al. (Eds.): HealthyIoT 2020, LNICST 360, pp. 77–92, 2021.
https://doi.org/10.1007/978-3-030-69963-5_6

about possible behavioral changes to improve the user's mental health and well-ness. The accumulated data can also contribute as a diagnostic measurement to detect early signs of changes to the user's cognitive health [19].

This paper extends from this idea of cognitive health tracking and considers how humans can use a wearable EEG device as a reliable and accessible eye health monitoring device. By placing EEG electrodes at certain positions on the scalp, users can gather cognitive activity data of particular interest. One such cognitive activity is the visual perception of the human eye, which directly connects to the brain through the visual cortex. Visually-evoked potentials (VEPs) correspond directly to the eye's visual acuity since VEPs are a measure of visual activity originating from the photoreceptors to the occipital cortex [9,34].

Visual acuity refers to how well the human eyes can precisely acquire details at a distance. This ability is quite complex, with many biological parts required to be in working order to process information [20]. Deficiencies in visual acuity have been shown to significantly reduce a person's quality of life [3,33]. Despite this importance, data collection to further understand and diagnose human vision is done through subject testimony, cellular response activation, or brain-based imaging techniques [4,35]. Personal testimonies are often subjective but widely used, for example, in the case of eye examinations. On the other hand, cellular responses and traditional non-wearable neuroimaging devices require substantial investment to procure and use [21,29,30].

This paper investigates how a wearable EEG device and a visual activity measurement technique known as steady-state visually evoked potential (SSVEP) can provide insight into the visual acuity of the human eye and hence human visual perception. Essentially, this study aims to quantify and perceive how the human eye sees.

### 1.1   Steady-State Visually Evoked Potential (SSVEP)

Steady-state visually evoked potentials are periodic responses evoked by a visual stimulus flickering at specific frequencies ranging from 1 to 90 Hz [16,30,31]. SSVEP responses oscillate at the same frequency as the flickering stimulus. SSVEP responses peak 15 Hz and decreases at higher frequencies [32]. EEG or functional magnetic resonance imaging (fMRI) can monitor SSVEP responses by measuring brain activation in the visual cortex [17,30].

### 1.2   Human Visual Perception

The human eye can see objects that emit or reflect light. The distance, spatial location, and the illuminance of the object affect perception. The density of receptor and ganglion cells in the retina is higher at the foveal area, and therefore central vision is more sensitive to observing details than the peripheral vision [37].

Varying levels of human attention impacts human visual perception [2]. A higher attention span has the effect of increasing SSVEP strength when a flickering stimulus is presented in the attended region of the visual field [6].

# 2    Ayinography

Ayinography is a technique to visualize the biological veillance flux of the human visual field by using the eye itself as a camera [11,24,25,27]. The participant is fitted with a wearable EEG sensing device, such as the Muse by Interaxon Inc. Normally, the Muse wearable device can only measure EEG signals at the frontal and temporal regions. By adding an external electrode, the device can detect EEG signals at the occipital point, the Oz location of the 10–20 system [18].

The ayinography technique requires the user to fix their eyes on a particular location while a stimulus traverses across the participant's visual field in a grid-like fashion. The wearable device records EEG data and obtains the SSVEP responses at every grid point location. These response activation values are mapped onto their corresponding spatial positions. This process repeats at varying distances from the user to construct a map of human visual perception. This study uses two different types of ayinography, a hardware-based and a software-based approach to prove the concept and investigate the human visual field as shown in Fig. 1.

## 2.1    Hardware Ayinography

The typical implementation of hardware-based ayinography utilizes the Sequential Wave Imprinting Machine (SWIM) technique to overlay the visual field onto the desired spatial plane. The SWIM uses multi-mediated reality to visualize invisible physical phenomenology, and thus it can be used for scientific measurement and analysis [7,10,22,23,26,28]. Typically, the SWIM uses a linear array of light sources connected to and receiving signals from a computing device. The array of light sources is moved back and forth to visualize measurements of waveforms. The system makes use of metavision, which is defined as the vision of vision [11], and overlays the human visual field onto the environment using augmented reality (AR).

Figure 1a shows an example of the hardware ayinography apparatus. The apparatus operates using two stepper motors and a belt assembly to move an arm in two dimensions within the bounds of its operation. The arm connects to a display device with a flashing stimulus at a set frequency. The plotter receives position vectors at regular intervals as the stimulus flashes. The user focuses on the approximate center of the apparatus as the stimulus traverses through the different predefined positions. Once the system collects the EEG data for all the predefined points, it constructs a mapping of the visual field of the mind's eye. The apparatus is then fitted with an RGB LED to trace out the mapping of the visual field. As the LED traverses, different colors are produced depending on the strength of the SSVEP response at a given position. The obtained result is a two-dimensional AR ayinograph by capturing the entire LED tracing process with a long-exposure photograph.

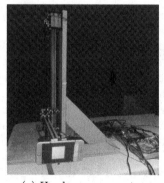    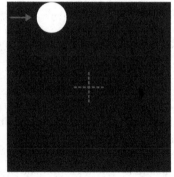

(a) Hardware apparatus.        (b) Software screen display.

**Fig. 1.** The hardware ayinography apparatus and the software ayinography display. (a) A display device with a flickering stimulus is secured to a robotic arm. The arm moves in a grid-like fashion, allowing for the collection of data to create the ayinograph. (b) An application which displays a flickering stimulus moving in a grid-like fashion to gather the data for vismaps required to create a software-based ayinograph. The red arrow shows the movement direction of the stimulus and the red cross shows the location of the center screen 3-pixel indicator. Both the red arrow and cross are visual aid overlays. (Color figure online)

### 2.2 Software Ayinography

The software ayinography makes use of a computer monitor as a two-dimensional plane as shown in Fig. 1b. The user focuses on a fixed graticule in the center of a black background while a stimulus of constant size flashes across the screen, traveling in a right-to-left and top-to-bottom manner. At each position, the stimulus flashes at a particular frequency for a fixed duration. Each position has 80 % overlap to the next known position. Once the EEG data is collected, the subsequent SSVEP activation mapping of the mind's eye results in a $23 \times 23 \, px$ slice of the user's visual field. The resulting representation is referred to as a vismap (or vidmap) from the Latin words "*visio*" which means "vision" (or "videre" which means "to see") and "*mappa*" which means a plane surface on which maps were drawn. The sequence may be repeated at various distances to the eye to recreate a three-dimensional ayinograph. Thus, software ayinography creates a more holistic mapping of the visual field through the mind's eye in three-dimensional space.

## 3    Signal Processing Algorithm

### 3.1    Lock-In Amplifier (LIA) Algorithm

The lock-in amplifier is originally an analog device that isolates and amplifies a certain oscillatory frequency while rejecting all other frequencies. This method of signal extraction is useful in an extremely noisy environment, provided that the reference signal frequency is precise and known. A more advanced form of LIA uses an additional reference signal that is 90° phase-shifted compared to the first reference. From Eq. 1, if the original reference is a cosine wave with a frequency set at $f_s$, then the additional reference is a sine wave.

$$sin(\omega t) = cos(\omega t + \frac{\pi}{2}), t = (t_1, t_2, \ldots, t_n)$$
$$\omega = 2\pi f_s$$

(1)

Given the frequency that the stimulus is flashing at, two reference signals, a sine wave and a cosine wave, are multiplied to the original signal. A software-based LIA is useful for the study since the algorithm extracts the SSVEP response frequency, as long as the stimulus frequency is known.

The algorithm replicates the performance of a hardware-based LIA. Eq. 2 details this implementation. The algorithm multiplies the raw 256 Hz sampled EEG data collected from the Oz position with the cosine and sine reference waves at the stimulus frequency to extract the SSVEP at that frequency. Then, a second-order Butterworth low-pass filter (LPF) at 0.7 Hz is applied to yield an output that mostly contains the amplitude information of the signal. The low-pass filter is set to 0.7 Hz since this is approximately a decade less than the frequencies of interest.

$$V_{cos}(\omega t_j) = \text{LPF}\left[u(t)cos(\omega t_j), 0.7\,\text{Hz}\right]$$
$$V_{sin}(\omega t_j) = \text{LPF}\left[u(t)sin(\omega t_j), 0.7\,\text{Hz}\right]$$
$$\alpha(\omega t_j) = \sqrt{V_{cos}(\omega t_j)^2 + V_{sin}(\omega t_j)^2}$$

(2)

Equation 3 averages the summed magnitudes, and this value indicates the extracted value of a particular spatial location.

$$pixel = \frac{1}{n}\sum_{j=1}^{n}\alpha(\omega t_j)$$

(3)

### 3.2   Threshold Denoising Algorithm

A simple threshold denoising algorithm is applied to isolate quantifiable features on the resulting bitmap. The algorithm weakens values below the threshold and strengthens the values above it. Next, by comparing each pixel value to its neighboring pixels and removing outliers, the single-pixel noise is removed. Lastly, the method averages the pixel value among the neighboring pixels by applying a Gaussian filter to the image.

## 4   Experimental Procedure

There were five participants in the experiments, 4 males and 1 female in their mid-20s to early 30s. All participants are not diagnosed with any brain or vision-related issues. User C and D wore prescription corrective lenses during the experiments. Table 1 lists the software ayinography experiment variation for each user.

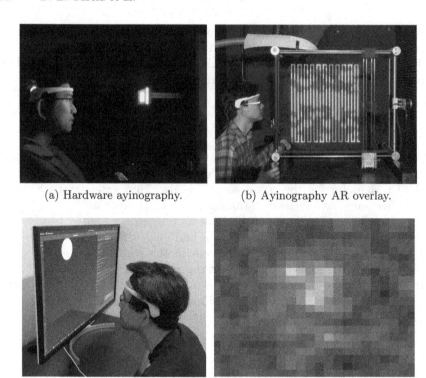

(a) Hardware ayinography.      (b) Ayinography AR overlay.

(c) Software ayinography.      (d) Vismap for 20 cm distance.

**Fig. 2.** A user participating in both software and hardware variants of the ayinography experiment. From left to right, the first image is the hardware ayinography experiment performed by a user. The second image is the hardware ayinograph overlayed onto the real-world environment using long-exposure photography at 8.5 Hz stimulus frequency and 2 s stimulus duration. The third image is the software ayinography experiment performed by the same user. The last image is the user's vismap at 20 cm, 8.5 Hz stimulus frequency and 2 s stimulus duration.

**Table 1.** Software ayinography experiment variation.

| User | Diagonal window size (cm) | Frequencies (Hz) |
|------|---------------------------|------------------|
| A | 43.5 | 6, 11, 16 |
| B | 26.8 | 7, 12, 17 |
| C | 53.0 | 8, 13, 18 |
| D | 38.1 | 9, 14, 19 |
| E | 22.5 | 10, 15, 20 |

Figure 2 shows a user performing the hardware and software experiments and their corresponding processed outputs. During the experiments, the users focus their vision on a centered indicator while the stimulus moves to different predefined locations. Table 1 summarizes, for each user, the frequency at which the stimulus flashes and the diagonal window size. Adding timestamps to both the collected EEG data and the stimulus position helps in matching the data to its corresponding position. At each predefined location, the stimulus flashes for a set duration of 1 s or 2 s for the software ayinography, and 2 s for the hardware ayinography experiment.

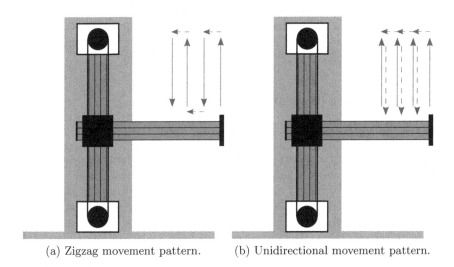

(a) Zigzag movement pattern.     (b) Unidirectional movement pattern.

**Fig. 3.** Side view of the hardware ayinography apparatus as the stimulus is being presented. The stimulus moves in the direction of the arrows and experiment proper occurs when the arrow is solid. Two different stimulus movement patterns are examined. (a) shows the zigzag movement pattern. (b) shows the unidirectional movement pattern.

In the software ayinography experiment, the stimulus moves left to right for each predefined row, and then top to bottom. The stimulus used is a $200 \times 200$ px black and white flashing circle. The stimulus size is dependent on the user's screen size, which is shown in Table 1. This experimental procedure mirrors a previous study investigating the SSVEP response with the stimulus at different positions [11]. Expanding from the previous study, the experiment is repeated with the user's eyes set at 20 cm, 30 cm, 40 cm, and 50 cm away from the screen to obtain enough data to reconstruct the user's field of vision.

In the hardware ayinography experiment, a square stimulus is projected using a smartphone with a screen size of 12 cm. This study experiments with two different stimulus movements as shown in Fig. 3. The first is a zigzag pattern where the stimulus moves from bottom to top, then back, and repeats in this fashion until the end of the experiment. The second is a unidirectional pattern where the stimulus starts from bottom to top and then resets to the next bottom position.

Once all the data are collected, the signals are processed using the software-defined lock-in amplifier (LIA) algorithm to extract the SSVEP at that frequency. The algorithm obtains the pixel value for each stimulus location by averaging the magnitude over the time duration for that particular stimulus location.

The vismaps that form the software ayinographs are generated by taking these averaged magnitudes and plotting them onto a heatmap based on their values. The threshold denoising algorithm is then applied to the vismaps to extract quantifiable information. The hardware ayinographs are formed by constructing a bitmap of the averaged magnitudes, scaling up to $42 \times 22$ px, and plotting the results with an RGB LED. Figure 2b shows a sample result as an augmented reality overlay using long-exposure photography.

## 5   Results and Discussion

### 5.1   Foveal Activation and Direction

Based on the results from software-based ayinography, the vismaps portrayed the existence of a foveal area through the mind's eye. This foveal area had a higher SSVEP activation, forming a circular pattern within the participant's field of view and corresponded to a higher intensity color as shown from the ayinographs in Fig. 4. The algorithm extracted this area by applying a threshold filter on the vismaps to remove noise. Certain images had high, isolated activations outside the foveal region. These outliers were then smoothed or dampened using the threshold denoising algorithm to increase the gains of the focal center. Figure 5 shows sample denoised vismaps that clearly show the focal center. The isolated focal center pixels were then computed and normalized by the window sizes, Table 1, used by each user. Figure 6 shows the retrieved foveal areas. For results in which a clear foveal area is not visible, the results are recorded as 0 px.

In both hardware and software ayinography, the SSVEP response peaked when the stimulus was flashing close to the central vision: the focal point. The foveal area was found to depend on stimulus distance, size, and duration. In the software ayinography, the focal point is represented by a circle of high activation in the center of vismaps, as shown in Fig. 4. In the hardware ayinography, the focal point is represented by lines of high activation near the center of the SWIM, as shown in Fig. 7.

Using these ayinography methods, a participant's focal point and attention could be visibly seen. In Fig. 7a, the participant was looking at a downward angle when the hardware ayinograph was taken, while in Fig. 7b, the same participant was looking straight.

From Fig. 6, as well as the original vismaps, data taken at 1 s stimulus duration had a higher rate of noise in the foveal area data compared to data taken at 2 s stimulus duration. Since the higher stimulus duration had more sample

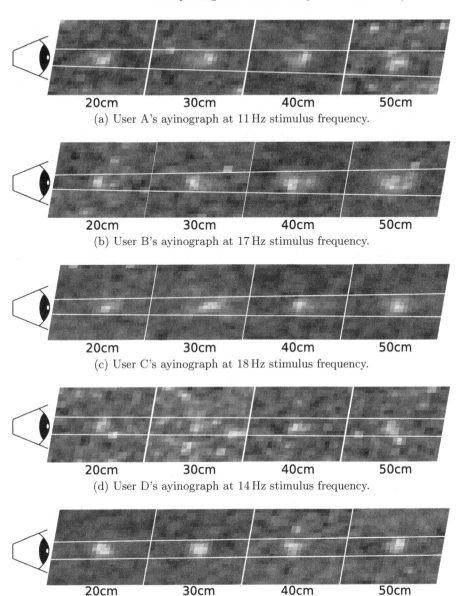

(a) User A's ayinograph at 11 Hz stimulus frequency.

(b) User B's ayinograph at 17 Hz stimulus frequency.

(c) User C's ayinograph at 18 Hz stimulus frequency.

(d) User D's ayinograph at 14 Hz stimulus frequency.

(e) User E's ayinograph at 15 Hz stimulus frequency.

**Fig. 4.** Software ayinograph obtained from each user's EEG data at 2 s stimulus duration. Vismaps at different distances are collated to form the ayinograph.

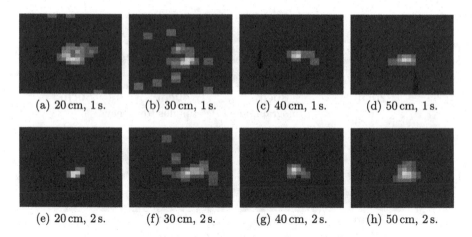

**Fig. 5.** Denoising of vismaps from User C at 18 Hz stimulus frequency in order to isolate the pixels for calculating the focal area. (a) to (d) are vismaps at 1 s stimulus duration. (e) to (h) are vismaps at 2 s stimulus duration.

points per stimulus location, the LIA algorithm has more data to work with for signal extraction and noise filtering.

Another observation was that the foveal area remained relatively static, with only a slightly increasing trend over the set of distances as shown in Fig. 4 and 7. Also, the foveal area changed for every stimulus frequency. Each user had a specific frequency which provided a consistently larger activation area: 11 Hz for User A, 17 Hz for User B, 13 Hz for User C, 9 Hz for User D, and 15 Hz for User E.

Subjects noted that the procedures were harder to follow for the hardware ayinography experiment than for software ayinography. The difficulty was due to the absence of a display that is coplanar to the stimulus. Subjects are required to refocus their vision whenever the stimulus enters and leaves their central field. Unfocusing and refocusing many times may cause changes in their attention levels and reconfigure their line of sight, which may decrease the SSVEP response strength.

## 5.2   Blink Interference

A human blink occurs at frequencies of 6 Hz and lower and strongly affects human visual perception and EEG signals [13]. Blinking affects visual perception since the individual momentarily loses sight of the stimulus while the eyes are closed. The muscle signals sent to the eye during a blink will interfere with SSVEP. The EEG amplifier will pick up this muscle signal as noise. This could have resulted in noisy data obtained at the 6 Hz by User A in Fig. 6a.

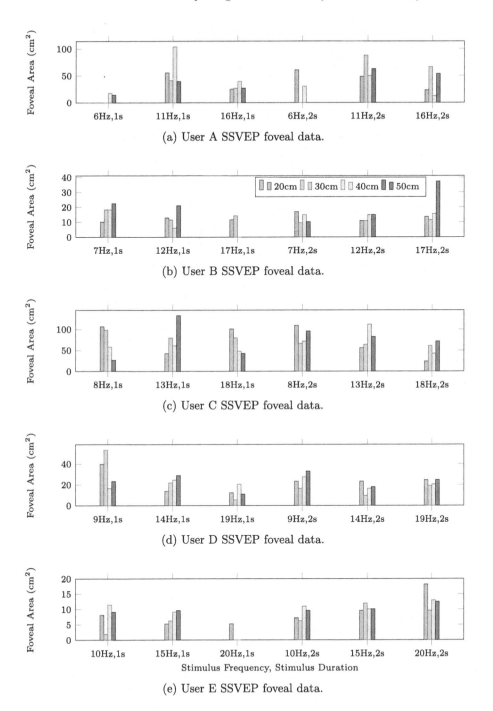

**Fig. 6.** Foveal area in cm² calculated based on SSVEP responses at various stimulus frequencies, duration and distance for each user.

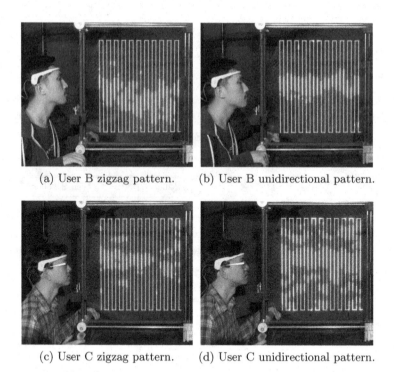

(a) User B zigzag pattern.          (b) User B unidirectional pattern.

(c) User C zigzag pattern.          (d) User C unidirectional pattern.

**Fig. 7.** Hardware ayinograph AR images from processed EEG data. (a) and (c) data are collected using a zigzag pattern while (b) and (d) are collected using the unidirectional pattern. Stimulus frequency for User B is set at 17 Hz while User C is set at 18 Hz. Stimulus duration for all experiments is set at 2 s.

## 5.3    SSVEP Response Delay

A response delay between the time of presentation of visual stimulus and the activation of SSVEP was examined during the experiments. This was clearly shown by comparing the results of the two moving patterns of hardware ayinography as seen in Fig. 7. When the stimulus was moving in a zigzag pattern, SSVEP response was shifted up and down depending on the direction of stimulus movement. In contrast, when the stimulus was moving in the unidirectional pattern, the start positions of the activations were more aligned. These contrasting observations indicate that the SSVEP activations were shifted in the same direction for the unidirectional pattern ayinographs.

As a result of the unidirectional shift, the area of activation in unidirectional pattern ayinographs had inherent inaccuracies since estimating the response time and the length of the shift were difficult. The response time in the zigzag pattern ayinographs shifted activation to both directions, minimizing the effect of response time on focal area estimations. Assuming response time is roughly the same for each row since activation on every other row is shifted in a different direction, the actual time for stimulus flashing is approximately the average of rows.

# 6   Conclusion

This paper provides an exploration of SSVEP frequencies, human vision, and response times. Wearable EEG devices can do more than just track users' sleep patterns, mental states, and cognitive health. Through the use of ayinography, EEG devices can also examine the foveal area of the human eye. This opens a potential path to personal eye informatics, perceiving and quantifying the visual acuity of the human eye.

Ayinography is a technique to visualize the visual field of the human as it changes in space. Two types of ayinography are presented: software-based and hardware-based. The software ayinograph is constructed with multiple vismaps at various distances. Each vismap represents the SSVEP responses obtained by displaying a moving flickering stimulus at a set distance from the eye. The hardware ayinograph is a two-dimensional AR overlay that is produced using long-exposure photography, and an LED tracing procedure to represent the SSVEP responses from a moving flickering stimulus.

Based on the results presented, the ayinography methods sufficiently capture the participant's focal point and attention. The foveal area remains largely static over distances, while a longer stimulus duration returns a less noisy signal for data collection. The existence of a response delay for SSVEP can be shown via the hardware ayinograph. The unidirectional pattern ayinograph shows a straight beam of activation from left to right, while the zigzag pattern ayinograph shows shifted activations based on the stimulus direction.

# 7   Future Work

## 7.1   Investigations into Stimulus Size

Due to the pandemic at the time of submission, experimental setups were recreated at multiple locations for each user. Thus, stimulus size, hardware specifications, and screen size were a few factors that had an effect on the outcome of the experiments. For future experiments, these factors may be explored or controlled.

## 7.2   Augmented Reality for Bioveillance

SWIMs, in general, have been used for visualizing phenomenological realities that are otherwise invisible to the human eye. By showing its usefulness in visualizing the human visual field, a future direction may include plans for using this augmented reality method to explore and visualize other biological phenomena.

## 7.3   Cognitive Studies and Visual Acuity

Ayinography can help determine the visual acuity of a person and quantify how eye defects hamper vision. This new form of visual perception analysis can lead to new insights into the correlations between vision and cognition. Additionally, using this technique, future directions can potentially lead to cognitive-visual exercises, brain-computer interfaces [12,24], or perhaps even explore visual perception within dreams.

## 7.4  Assessment Tool for Eye Health

Ayinography can be developed for use as an eye health assessment tool. When one visits the eye doctor, some degree of subjectivity in the form of user testimony is still present. Assessment by ayinography is more objective and accurate. By using a wearable EEG device, the assessment method becomes more accessible and cost-effective both in terms of assessment time and economic costs over traditional non-wearable neuroimaging devices. Using different colors in the flashing stimulus may provide insight into the presence of color blindness.

**Acknowledgements.** Special thanks to Jesse Hernandez for his valuable advice, opinions, and assistance with the project. The authors also thank other members of MannLab Canada for their continued support.

# References

1. Bietz, M.J., Hayes, G.R., Morris, M.E., Patterson, H., Stark, L.: Creating meaning in a world of quantified selves. IEEE Pervasive Comput. **15**(2), 82–85 (2016)
2. Boynton, G.M.: Attention and visual perception. Curr. Opin. Neurobiol. **15**(4), 465–469 (2005)
3. Brown, G.C.: Vision and quality-of-life. Trans. Am. Ophthalmol. Soc. **97**, 473 (1999)
4. Cao, D., Nicandro, N., Barrionuevo, P.A.: A five-primary photostimulator suitable for studying intrinsically photosensitive retinal ganglion cell functions in humans. J. Vis. **15**(1), 27 (2015)
5. Casson, A.J., Yates, D.C., Smith, S.J.M., Duncan, J.S., Rodriguez-Villegas, E.: Wearable electroencephalography. IEEE Eng. Med. Biol. Mag. **29**(3), 44–56 (2010)
6. Ding, J., Sperling, G., Srinivasan, R.: Attentional modulation of SSVEP power depends on the network tagged by the flicker frequency. Cereb. Cortex **16**(7), 1016–1029 (2006)
7. Do, P.V., Garcia, D.E., Lu, Z., Hernandez, J., Mann, S.: Steady-state visually-evoked potentials and sequential wave imprinting machine. In: IEEE International Conference on Systems, Man, and Cybernetics (SMC), Toronto, Ontario. IEEE (2020, in Press)
8. Dobbins, C., Rawassizadeh, R.: Clustering of physical activities for quantified self and mhealth applications. In: 2015 IEEE International Conference on Computer and Information Technology; Ubiquitous Computing and Communications; Dependable, Autonomic and Secure Computing; Pervasive Intelligence and Computing, Liverpool, UK, pp. 1423–1428. IEEE (2015)
9. Dustman, R.E., et al.: Age and fitness effects on EEG, ERPs, visual sensitivity, and cognition. Neurobiol. Aging **11**(3), 193–200 (1990)

10. Garcia, D.E., Mertens, A., Hernandez, J., Li, M., Mann, S.: HDR (high dynamic range) audio wearable and its performance visualization. In: IEEE International Conference on Systems, Man, and Cybernetics (SMC), Toronto, Ontario. IEEE (2020, in Press)
11. Garcia, D.E., Zheng, K.W., Liu, Y., Tao, Y.S., Mann, S.: Painting with the eye: understanding the visual field of the human eye with SSVEP. In: IEEE International Conference on Systems, Man, and Cybernetics (SMC), Toronto, Ontario. IEEE (2020, in Press)
12. Garcia, D.E., Zheng, K.W., Tao, Y.S., Liu, Y., Mann, S.: Capturing pictures from human vision using SSVEP and lock-in amplifier. In: 33rd Conference on Graphics, Patterns and Images, Porto de Galinhas, Brazil. IEEE (2020, submitted)
13. Gasser, T., Sroka, L., Möcks, J.: The transfer of EOG activity into the EEG for eyes open and closed. Electroencephalogr. Clin. Neurophysiol. Suppl. **61**(2), 181–193 (1985)
14. Gilmore, J.N.: Everywear: the quantified self and wearable fitness technologies. New Media Soc. **18**(11), 2524–2539 (2016)
15. Haddadi, H., Ofli, F., Mejova, Y., Weber, I., Srivastava, J.: 360-degree quantified self. In: 2015 International Conference on Healthcare Informatics, Dallas, TX, USA, pp. 587–592. IEEE (2015)
16. Herrmann, C.S.: Human EEG responses to 1–100 Hz flicker: resonance phenomena in visual cortex and their potential correlation to cognitive phenomena. Exp. Brain Res. **137**(3–4), 346–353 (2001). https://doi.org/10.1007/s002210100682
17. Hillyard, S.A., et al.: Combining steady-state visual evoked potentials and fMRI to localize brain activity during selective attention. Hum. Brain Mapp. **5**(4), 287–292 (1997). https://doi.org/10.1002/(sici)1097-0193(1997)5:4⟨287::aid-hbm14⟩3.0.co;2-b
18. Jasper, H.: Report of the committee on methods of clinical examination in electroencephalography. Electroencephalogr. Clin. Neurophysiol. **10**, 370–375 (1958)
19. Kunze, K., Iwamura, M., Kise, K., Uchida, S., Omachi, S.: Activity recognition for the mind: toward a cognitive "quantified self". Computer **46**(10), 105–108 (2013)
20. Lit, A.: Visual acuity. Annu. Rev. Psychol. **19**(1), 27–54 (1968)
21. Lovie-Kitchin, J.E.: Validity and reliability of visual acuity measurements. Ophthalmic Physiol. Opt. **8**(4), 363–370 (1988)
22. Mann, S., Do, P.V., Lu, Z., Lau, J.K.K.: Sequential wave imprinting machine (SWIM) implementation using SDR (software-defined radio). In: 2020 Seventh International Conference on Software Defined Systems (SDS), Paris, France, pp. 123–130. IEEE (2020)
23. Mann, S.: Phenomenological augmented reality with the sequential wave imprinting machine (SWIM). In: 2018 IEEE Games, Entertainment, Media Conference (GEM), Galway, Ireland, pp. 1–9. IEEE (2018)
24. Mann, S., et al.: Encephalogames TM (brain/mind games): inclusive health and wellbeing for people of all abilities. In: 2019 IEEE Games, Entertainment, Media Conference (GEM), New Haven, CT, USA, pp. 1–10. IEEE (2019)
25. Mann, S., et al.: Keynote-eye itself as a camera: sensors, integrity, and trust. In: The 5th ACM Workshop on Wearable Systems and Applications, pp. 1–2. ACM, New York (2019)
26. Mann, S., Do, P.V., Garcia, D.E., Hernandez, J., Khokhar, H.: Electrical engineering design with the subconscious mind. In: 2020 IEEE International Conference on Human-Machine Systems (ICHMS), pp. 1–6. IEEE (2020)

27. Mann, S., et al.: Wearable computing, 3D aug* reality, photographic/videographic gesture sensing, and veillance. In: Proceedings of the Ninth International Conference on Tangible, Embedded, and Embodied Interaction, pp. 497–500. ACM, New York (2015)
28. Mann, S., Garcia, D.E., Do, P.V., Lam, D., Scourboutakos, P.: Visualizing electric machines with sequential wave imprinting machine. In: 22nd Symposium on Virtual and Augmented Reality (SVR), Porto de Galinhas, Brazil. IEEE (2020, in Press)
29. Mihajlović, V., Grundlehner, B., Vullers, R., Penders, J.: Wearable, wireless EEG solutions in daily life applications: what are we missing? IEEE J. Biomed. Health Inform. 19(1), 6–21 (2014)
30. Norcia, A.M., Appelbaum, L.G., Ales, J.M., Cottereau, B.R., Rossion, B.: The steady-state visual evoked potential in vision research: a review. J. Vis. 15(6), 4 (2015)
31. Panicker, R.C., Puthusserypady, S., Sun, Y.: An asynchronous P300 BCI with SSVEP-based control state detection. IEEE Trans. Biomed. Eng. 58(6), 1781–1788 (2011). https://doi.org/10.1109/tbme.2011.2116018
32. Pastor, M.A., Artieda, J., Arbizu, J., Valencia, M., Masdeu, J.C.: Human cerebral activation during steady-state visual-evoked responses. J. Neurosci. 23(37), 11621–11627 (2003). https://doi.org/10.1523/jneurosci.23-37-11621.2003
33. Rahi, J.S., Cumberland, P.M., Peckham, C.S.: Visual impairment and vision-related quality of life in working-age adults: findings in the 1958 British birth cohort. Ophthalmology 116(2), 270–274 (2009)
34. Sokol, S.: Visually evoked potentials: theory, techniques and clinical applications. Survey Ophthalmol. 21(1), 18–44 (1976)
35. Sue, S.: Test distance vision using a Snellen chart. Commun. Eye Health 20(63), 52 (2007)
36. Swan, M.: The quantified self: fundamental disruption in big data science and biological discovery. Big Data 1(2), 85–99 (2013)
37. Wandell, B., Thomas, S.: Foundations of vision. Psyccritiques 42(7), 649 (1997)

# Psychological Data Tracking Wearables, Applications and Systems

# Stress Detection with Deep Learning Approaches Using Physiological Signals

Fabrizio Albertetti[1], Alena Simalastar[2], and Aïcha Rizzotti-Kaddouri[1(✉)]

[1] School of Engineering, Haute Ecole Arc Ingénierie, Neuchatel, Switzerland
{fabrizio.albertetti,aicha.rizzotti}@he-arc.ch
[2] School of Engineering, Haute Ecole Spécialisée Valais-Wallis, Sion, Switzerland
alena.simalatsar@hevs.ch

**Abstract.** The problem of stress detection and classification has attracted a lot of attention in the past decade. It has been tackled with mainly two different approaches, where signals were either collected in ambulatory settings, which can be limited to the period of presence in the hospital, or in continuous mode in the field. A sensor-based continuous measurement of stress in daily life has a potential to increase awareness of patterns of stress occurrence. In this work, we first present a data-flow infrastructure suitable for two types of studies that conforms with the data protection requirements of the ethics committee monitoring the research on humans. The detection and binary classification of stress events is compared with three different machine learning models based on the features (meta-data) extracted from physiological signals acquired in laboratory conditions and ground-truth stress level information provided by the subjects themselves via questionnaires associated with these features. The main signals considered in current classification are electro-dermal activity (EDA) and blood volume pulse (BVP) signals. Different models are compared and the best configuration yields an $F_1$ score of 0.71 (random baseline: 0.48). The importance on prediction of phasic and tonic EDA components is also investigated. Our results also pave the way for further work on this topic with both machine learning approaches and signal processing directions.

**Keywords:** Physiological monitoring · Stress prediction · Sympathetic and parasympathetic activation · Affective computing · Telemonitoring · Self-management systems

## 1 Introduction

At the physiological level, stress is an organism's response to some external stimuli, or a challenge. In presence of stressor, the "fight or flight" response is

This project is funded by the University of Applied Sciences and Arts of Western Switzerland.

F. Albertetti and A. Simalastar—Both authors contributed equally to this paper.

© ICST Institute for Computer Sciences, Social Informatics and Telecommunications Engineering 2021
Published by Springer Nature Switzerland AG 2021. All Rights Reserved
R. Goleva et al. (Eds.): HealthyIoT 2020, LNICST 360, pp. 95–111, 2021.
https://doi.org/10.1007/978-3-030-69963-5_7

activated through the sympathetic nervous system (SNS), which results in release of cortisol and adrenaline, leading to heart rate increase, sweating, and increased concentration of all senses on current situation. The parasympathetic nervous system (PSNS) works in concert with SNS. Its main function is to activate the 'rest and digest' response and return the body to homeostasis after the "fight or flight" response. This results in a reversion of the physical effects of SNS activation and particularly in a heart-rate decrease. Both SNS and PSNS represent the autonomous nervous system (ANS).

In a sense, stress is a natural reaction of the organism. However, there exist many studies showing the link between stress and illnesses [18]. This means that it is not the fact of stress that causes problems to the organism, it is the level of stress that might be excessive to an organism, such that the PSNS fails to return it to homeostasis. Such an excessive and often prolonged stress is called a *distress*. Identification of distress is not simple, since asking a person about how she or he thinks, or feel is susceptible to a wide range of biases since humans are very often not even aware of how they are affected by various stimuli or situations. This way, it is important to give an objective quantitative evaluation to the level of stress and study the activation of ANS as the first step towards definition of the border between a positive stimulation of the organism and distress. This may allow to not only detect the stress conditions leading to distress, but potentially reduce the fear of stress and its unnecessary consequences.

The approaches to stress detection can be roughly classified into: 1) those performed in the ambulatory setting during a relatively short period of time, and 2) those that are performed during the long term when the participant continue his/her normal life activities. The signals reflecting the ANS activity, can be divided into *physiological*, such as, for example, electro-dermal activity (EDA) [4], heart rate (HR), heart rate variability (HRV) [15], and levels of cortisol [13,20], and *behavioural*, such as smartphone activity statistics [16], and annotated geolocation. It is clear that experiment settings define the set of signals that must be considered as more reliable for that experiment. It is obvious that *behavioural* signals make much less sense in the ambulatory settings as well as the level of cortisol, since its level is a subject to circadian rhythms. The other *physiological* signals (EDA, HR, and HRV), in contrast, are less reliable in long terms studies since they are often heavily corrupted with the movement artifacts that are difficult to filter out. However, their good classification in the laboratory setting could help to find the means to improve their use in the long term studies.

The ultimate goal of our study is a system for real-life seamless monitoring of stress. Therefore, we have first created a data-flow application suitable for two types of studies that conforms with the data protection requirements of the ethics committee monitoring the research on humans, as described in this paper.

The stress classification approach presented in this paper is covering the experiments performed in the laboratory setting during which EDA, and HRV signals were collected by means of the Empatica E4 wrist bracelet. The participants of the experiment were induced with four types of stress stimuli, aiming to provoke *emotional*, *intellectual*, and *physical activity* types of stress as well as *pain*, alternated with relaxation periods. The signals are annotated with the indicators of relative changes of perceived stress levels provided by each participant. Further, all the signals are processed and vectors of important signals features are extracted. The vectors of signal features with stress indicators are then combined into simple or multiple windows and given as an input to machine learning based models. Furthermore, a comparison of deep learning models is presented.

This paper is organized as follows: Sect. 2 presents related work for stress evaluation, Sect. 3 provides details on the dataset, Sect. 4 presents details of each data-flow step and Sect. 5 discuss experimental results. Finally, in Sect. 6 we summarize the importance of our contribution and suggest some future work.

## 2 Related Work

Several works proposed in literature aim to detect the condition of stress and estimate the level of mental effort by using wearable sensors and mobile applications, such as in [3] and [12], which have demonstrated that smartphone data can be used for mood classification.

Physiological measures such as EDA, HR and HRV are frequently used in studies related to affection and well-being [16]. [6] proposes a smart-watch based system to collect and analyses biosignal data to detect unobtrusively and at low cost mental stress condition during daily life activities. In particular, EDA has long been used to study a variety of physiological subjects including stress, emotion, depression, anxiety, attention and information processing [7]. In [16] the link between EDA and stress is explored. In the same study, the authors collected data for the analysis and prediction of stress from smartphone logs. [14] proves that the EDA is sensitive to cognitive stress during water immersion while others used derivatives of the BVP signal as in [9] where information on respiratory rate (RR) and HRV is analyzed to obtain reliable interpretation parameters for stress assessment.

Some works have also added other types of data to better support their results as in [2] which adds diameter of the pupil to the characteristics of the user's physiological signals such as blood volume pulse (BVP) providing HRV, galvanic skin response (GSR), i.e. EDA, and temperature of the skin, to provide a system for detecting stress. In [10], a classification method to determine stress on GSR and speech was proposed. In our work we are focusing on signals that can be acquired in a seamless manned in everyday life. Therefore, we are not considering pupil dilatation as a potential physiological measure for our system, even though we admit that it is a useful indicator of stress. Though, we might consider speech recognition as a potential extension of our system in the future.

The wide variety of classification algorithms have been applied to tackle the classification problem. In [2], signal processing techniques were applied to the physiological signals monitored to extract characteristics used by various learning algorithms: Naive Bayes, decision trees, and SVM to classify relaxed states (non-stress) compared to stressed states (stress). In [10], the decision tree, K-means clustering, and support vector machine (SVM) classifiers were proposed. In [6] a

KNN classifier was used to predict stress, from the body temperature, GSR and RR interval. The signals were collected to detect mental stress generated by the subject solving the Tower of Hanoi puzzle. This work [21] used logistic regression to predict the probability of stress state. In [11], the authors use a deep learning model with 7 hidden layers to predict stress state using EEG signal. It is common to classify stress with a binary class as in [8], with an RNN algorithm detecting stress from a voice signal.

The most relevant to our approach is the method of WESAD experiment [17], during which a multi modal data set was collected for stress classification and tested by several algorithms based on physiological data. Data collection was carried out in the laboratory. A binary definition of stress (stress, non-stress), as well as a three-class definition (baseline, stress, and amusement), are tested. However, all the tested algorithms are based on single sequence inputs, such as decision trees, kNN, or AdaBoost.

## 3   Data Collection

In this section, we describe how the DESY dataset used for the detection and classification of stress was collected.

The signals were acquired from 6 students of our university who have signed the consent form. The study protocol (see Sect. 3.1) was approved by the ethics committee on human resource (CER-VD) [1]. Exclusion criteria, stated in the study invitation, were pregnancy or lactation, major psycho-neuro-endocrinological or cardiac diseases and mental disorders, as well as participants having insufficient knowledge of the project language. All selected subject wore the Empatica E4 bracelet on their non dominant hand and the E4 records BVP (64 Hz), EDA (4 Hz), TEMP (4 Hz), and ACC (32 Hz) were recorded during the whole study. For more details about collected signals see Sect. 4. All the collected data were carefully anonymized.

### 3.1   Study Protocol

The goal of this experiment was to record physiological signals that will have the least possible movement induced artifacts often corrupting the physiological data collected using wearable technologies. Therefore, this experiment was performed in the laboratory conditions, while the participants were asked to make as little as possible movement with the hand with the bracelet to avoid as much as possible the movement artifacts. As the possible sources of stress we have selected the *emotional arousal*, *intellectual efforts*, *physical exercises*, and *pain*.

In order to allow each participant to come to his/her baseline condition the experiment was started by filling in a small questionnaire that was used further to define the subjective level of the current health and stress conditions. The participants were asked to answer the following questions using the 5 grade-scale:

- In general, my health is... - *[Excellent (5) .. Poor (1)]*
- I feel energetic... - *[All of the time (5) .. Almost never (1)]*
- Personality: I often stress when unexpected and difficult situations arise - *[Strongly agree (5) .. Strongly disagree (1)]*
- Daily activities: I stressed a lot in the past 24 h - *[Strongly agree (5) .. Strongly disagree (1)]*
- Sleep quality (1): I had trouble sleeping and had many sleep disturbances last night - *[Strongly agree (5) .. Strongly disagree (1)]*
- Sleep quality (2): I did not sleep in the past 24 h - *[Strongly agree (5) .. Strongly disagree (1)]*
- Sleep quality (3): I had trouble sleeping and had many sleep disturbances in the past month - *[Strongly agree (5) .. Strongly disagree (1)]*
- Right now, I fell... - *[Relaxed (5) .. Stressed (1)]*

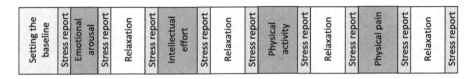

**Fig. 1.** An example of sequence of stressful and relaxing events with questionnaires. Note that each participant had his own order of stressful events.

To emulate each of the sources of stress each participant was asked to perform different activities. This way:

1. *Emotional arousal* was stimulated by showing a scary video during about 3 min;
2. *Intellectual efforts* was done by solving some riddles that were chosen by each participant randomly from a bunch of riddles printed on a paper (2–3 min);
3. *Physical activity* was represented by series of squats (2–3 min);
4. *Pain* was emulated by letting the participant to put his hand in the icy water for 1–2 min.

Each volunteer was participating in the above described studies with the randomized order of stress test to avoid influence of the order of stressful events on the results of classification. Each stressful period was followed by minimum 7 min of relaxation with some peaceful music and videos of the nature.

After each period (stressful or relaxed) of the experiment, each participate was asked to report their perceived stress level regarding the just finished activity describing it as either of the following: 1) I feel more relaxed, 2) No difference, 3) I feel less relaxed, and 4) I feel more stressed. An example of the sequence of stressful and relaxing events is shown on Fig. 1.

## 4    Methods

The general architecture of the dataflow in our data processing chain is presented on Fig. 2. It starts with the raw physiological signals collected from bracelet sensors (1), which are further sent to the mobile application (2). Next, the data flow is securely sent to the RedCap platform (3), frequently used and recommended for managing medical data. The data are stored in the cloud for further extraction of various features (4) using our proprietary signal processing and feature extraction algorithms. After signal processing, the features are sent back sent to the REDCap cloud. Further, the data are picked up by a classification algorithm (5) capable of predicting the stressful events (6).

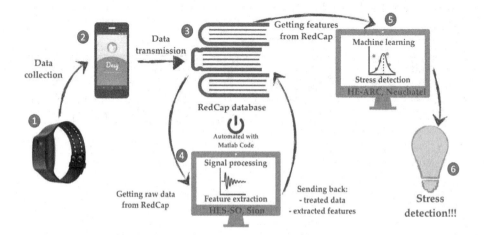

**Fig. 2.** The general architecture of the dataflow.

### 4.1    Wearable Sensor

The Empatica E4 bracelet[1], the device that was used for this work, offers the acquisition of physiological signals in real-time. The company has made available the Empatica Connect platform[2], which allows to visualise the graphs corresponding to the different signals. The bracelet works in two modes: (a) *streaming mode*: the bracelet connects via Bluetooth with the mobile application, and (b) *recording mode*: the wristband records the data in the internal memory, while it can record up to 60 h. The Empatica E4 bracelet is equipped with the following physiological sensors:

- EDA Sensor (or GSR Sensor): The skin is the only tissue of human body that is innervated by only SNS branches of the ANS and not by PNS branch fibres.

---

[1] https://www.empatica.com/en-eu/research/e4.
[2] https://www.empatica.com/connect.

Activation of the SNS provokes activation of sweat gland and thereby reducing skin electrical resistance and increasing conductance, whose fluctuating changes are measured by the EDA sensor in μSiemens. Consists of a tonic (referred to as skin conductance level (SCL)) and a phasic (skin conductance response (SCR)) component.

- PPG Sensor (Photoplethysmography Sensor) measures the blood volume pulse (BVP) from which two important signals can be derived: (1) heart rate (HR), and the inter-beat-interval (IBI). The blood volume pulse is measured in nanoWatts, heart rate HR in beats per minute (bpm), while IBI is measured in time periods between two consecutive beats.
- Infrared Thermopile: measures the temperature of the skin and contains the data measured in celsius degrees.
- 3-axis Accelerometer (ACC): measures activity based on motion, contains the data of the 3-axis channels (x, y, and z) accelerometer sensor. It measures continuous gravitational force (g) applied to each of the three spacial dimensions.

As was already mentioned earlier, in our study, we have used the signals acquired only with EDA and PPG sensors. We believe that skin temperature is greatly influenced by the temperature of the environment and therefore without knowing the real environmental conditions it would be difficult to receive a meaningful informations out of that particular signals. ACC signal, in contrast, is very useful, especially for classification of different types of stress, in particular differentiation between physical activity, with intensive movements or pain, with abrupt movement, and emotional/intellectual stress, with minimal movements. However, in this work we aim at binary classification, and therefore, the ACC signal is not used in the current study. Once we extend the use of our prediction model to the 5-class stress identification, this signal will be used.

## 4.2   Mobile Application

In order to perform experiments we have developed our proprietary mobile application for Android mobile platform with a user-friendly frontend and a backend performing three basic features, such as:

1. Data collection from the Empatica E4 bracelet and its temporal storage at the smartphone;
2. Questionnaire, allowing to collect the perceived level of stress by each participant;
3. Secure transmission of the recorded data into the RedCap database.

As temporary storage before sending data to cloud REDCap database at the end of each experiment an intern database (SQlite) was used. Once the experiment was over, all the signals were converted into the comma-separated values (CSV) format and were sent to the cloud for further processing.

### 4.3    REDCap Database

There exist several secure solutions to support human health data collection and storage. REDCap[3] is one of those with the further advantage of being available for free for research purposes. REDCap is a secure web application for building and managing online surveys and databases. REDCap provides multiple useful features, including secure mailing facilities supporting exchange of big data among researcher participants, as well as a built-in project calendar, a scheduling module, and ad hoc reporting tools. One feature of interest is the REDCap Mobile App interface that allows collecting data offline, for example, by a mobile device when there is no Wi-Fi or cellular connection, and then, later, sync data back to the server.

The logical portions of data in REDCap are grouped as 'Instruments'. The instruments of the DESY database in REDCap can be classified into communications with participants of the experiment (e.g. consent form), and 'instruments folders' containing raw signals, features extracted from the raw signals, and questionnaires, providing ground-truth information.

### 4.4    Signal Processing

Signal processing was automatized, such that in one click all the available signal processing techniques are performed on the raw data following the steps:

1. Getting the raw data from the REDCap;
2. Signal processing, analysis and restoration;
3. Features extraction;
4. Sending processed signals and features to REDCap.

It is quite often that the signals recorded by Empatica E4 bracelet are incomplete, such that some data are lost. This usually happens if the signal quality was not good enough, for example, due to the weak connection of the PPG sensor with the wrist. However, since feature extraction is done by small portions from a part of signal selected by a window of as parameterized size sliding over the signal with a regular step, it is crucial to have a complete signal. Therefore, we have developed several methods for restoration of lost data based on another available signal.

After analyzing the collected data, we have discovered that the most corrupted physiological signal among those collected from E4 is the BVP signal of the PPG sensor. However, it is rare that the data are lost from more than 20 s, especially when the experiments are performed in laboratory setting with minimum movements during the experiment. Therefore, first of all we have implemented an algorithm for HR signal extraction from BVP E4 signal by using a simple Fast Fourier Transform (FFT) for a sliding window size (i.e. 30 s, 1 min etc.) of the signal with a variable step that can be chosen according to the need, e.g. 1 s, 5 s, 30 s, etc.

---

[3] https://www.project-redcap.org/.

Apart from the raw BVP signal, Empatica E4 bracelet provides the IBI signal, the derivative of the BVP, representing the series of time interval between individual beats of the participant heart, largely used in the HRV analysis (see Sect. 4.5). Since IBI signal is build directly from the BVP signal that has missing data, it also has missing data in the same time periods. However, the reconstruction of IBI signal is simpler than of the raw BVP. Therefore, we have developed another algorithm that is reconstructing the missing parts of the IBI signal from the HR signal extracted using our first algorithm. Such a reconstruction cannot result in an ideal signal. Therefore, we also create a vector of quality of each value of the IBI time series with three quality levels, where level 0 corresponds to an optimal quality (the values provided by Empatica E4), level 2 - are the values reconstructed from the HR, and level 3 - values that have no meaning. Currently, this vector is not used but in our future work it is planned to be used by the classification algorithm to weight the credibility of the data.

### 4.5    Features Extracted

The main signals used for classification were the IBI and EDA. This section summarizes the features extracted from these two signals.

**HRV Analysis:** IBI signal analysis is often also called HRV analysis, and it is the study of variations in the instantaneous heart rate time series using the beat-to-beat RR-intervals (the RR tachogram, not to confuse with Respiratory Rate (RR)). There exist three main approaches to HRV analysis: 1) time-domain based, 2) frequency domain based, and 3) geometrical methods. The HR may be increased due to activation of the SNS or decreased due to PSNS (vagal) activity. While, in opposite, the variability of HR is decreasing with the activation of the SNS and increasing with PSNS, leading to the decrease (for SNS) and increase (for PSNS) of standard deviation (STD) of RR-intervals. The balance between the effects of SNS and PSNS, is called sympathovagal balance and is believed to be reflected in the beat-to-beat changes of the cardiac cycle. The time domain features (mostly various calculations of STD of RR-intervals) used in our study are presented in Table 1. While the frequency domain and geometrical domain features are presented in Table 2 and 3, respectively.

**Table 1.** Time domain features

| Feature | Formula |
|---|---|
| Standard deviation | $SDNN = \frac{1}{N-1}\sqrt{(\sum_{i=1}^{N}(RR_i - \overline{RR})^2)}$ |
| Coefficient of variation | $CV = \frac{SDNN}{RR}$ |
| Standard deviation of the average RR interval | $SDSD = \frac{1}{N-1}\sqrt{(\sum_{i=1}^{N-1}(\Delta RR_i - \overline{\Delta RR})^2)}$ <br> $\Delta RR_i = RR_{i+1} - RR_i$ |
| Mean difference of successive NN intervals | $RMSSD = \frac{1}{N-1}\sqrt{(\sum_{i=1}^{N-1}(RR_{i+1} - RR_i)^2)}$ |
| Number of RR intervals | $NN50$ |
| Vagus activity | $pNN50 = \frac{NN50}{(N-1)}$ |

**Table 2.** Frequency domain features

| Feature | Formula | Meaning |
|---------|---------|---------|
| The power of the complete signal | $TP$ | Associated with the hypothalamic-pituitary complex activity |
| High frequency 0.15–0.4 Hz | $HF$ | Associated with breathing arrhythmia and PSNS activity. Subject to circadian rhythms 24 h signal analyzed |
| Normalized HF | $nHF = HF/TP$ | |
| Low frequency 0.04–0.15 Hz | $LW$ | Slow waves of first order, SNS activity. Subject to circadian rhythms if 24 h signal analyzed |
| Normalized LF | $nLF = LF/TP$ | Grows with SNS activation, since TP goes down and LF does not change |
| Index of vagosympathetic cooperation | $LF/HF$ | |
| Very low frequency 0.015–0.04 Hz | $VLF$ | Psycho-emotional tension |
| Ultra low frequency <0.003 Hz | $ULF$ | Is measured only for long term signals ($\approx$24 h). Subject to circadian rhythm. Therefore, it was not used in our study |
| Index of centralization | $IC = (VLF + LF)/HF$ | |

**Table 3.** Geometrical domain features

| Feature | Formula |
|---------|---------|
| Mode of the histogram | $Mo$ |
| Amplitude of the histogram | $AMo$ |
| Width of the histogram | $Delta_X(TINN)$ |
| Width normalized value | $Dealta_X/RR$ |
| Index of SNS activity | $SNS_{ind} = AMo/(2 * Mo * delta_X)$ |
| Index of PSNS activity | $PSNS_{ind} = 1/(Mo * delta_X)$ |

**Table 4.** EDA time domain features

| Description | Feature |
|---|---|
| SCR amplitude peak counts | $EDA_{peakCount}$ |
| The minimum value found in the section | $EDA_{MIN}$ |
| The maximum value in the section | $EDA_{MAX}$ |
| Area under curve | $EDA_{AUC}$ |
| Mean of first order derivatives | $EDA_{MEAN\_derivative}$ |
| Mean of negative values of first order derivatives | $EDA_{MEAN\_negative\_derivative}$ |
| Hjorth features [19] | $EDA_{complexity}$ |

**EDA Analysis.** The overall signal called EDA of electrodermal activity consists of two components. One of the components is the EDA general tonic level which relates to an overall signal level, the most common measure of this component is the SCL and the changes in the SCL are believed to reflect the general changes in autonomic arousal. The value of SCL can vary widely, typically between 2–20 μS, due to environmental and personal factors [5]. The second component is the phasic component and this refers to the fast response variations of the signal in the form of peaks, i.e. the SCRs, and appears either in response to a stimulus or without evident stimulation. These instantaneous peaks can be characterized by a rise time, amplitude and a half recovery time. In healthy adults, the rise time is usually between 1 and 3 s, the amplitude often varies (a minimum is usually between 0.01 and 0.05 μS), and the half recovery time is usually between 2 and 10 s [5]. The example of an EDA signal annotated with stress stimuli is presented on Fig. 3.

From these signals we can extract several features in the time and frequency domain. For our study we have chosen the most relevant ones, that are presented in Tables 4 and 5.

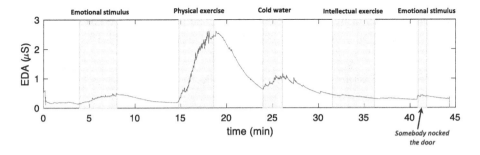

**Fig. 3.** The EDA signal with four stressful activities and an unexpected stressful even related to the knocking on the door.

**Table 5.** EDA frequency domain features

| Description | Formula |
|---|---|
| Energy of the signal | $EDA_{Signal\_Energy}$ |
| Summation of FFT harmonics | $EDA_{harmonics\_summation}$ |
| Area under curve of FFT | $EDA_{AUC\_fft}$ |
| Standard deviation of FFT | $EDA_{STD\_fft}$ |
| Mean of FFT | $EDA_{MEAN\_fft}$ |
| Signal values in the frequency domain | $EDA_{coefficients}$ |

## 4.6   Machine Learning

Stress can be detected and predicted by machine learning methods with classification or regression models. In the DESY dataset, stress and its predictors are represented as a time series.

For the purpose of binary classification, we decided to compare 3 different methods. First, a decision tree models based on a summarized time window is presented. Second, a recurrent neural network (RNN) capable of handling multiple time windows is tested. And third, an augmented RNN with some convolutional layers first (CRNNs) is tested for a more in-depth extraction of features.

**Architecture and Learning Process.** The DESY dataset consists of 6 patients, each with a duration of about 44 min. Due to the nature of time series and to the need of a stratified split, we used 4 patients for the training set and 2 patients for the test set, resulting in 28% for the test set, cross-validated (K = 3).

The stress label, as described in Sect. 3, is filled in by participants at the end of each period. All the values in between these periods are linearly interpolated. The decision tree is augmented with gradient boosting and implemented with the CatBoost library. The prediction of a single time window is performed with a maximum depth of 6. The RNN consists of a single layer of LSTM cells, some batch normalization, and a dense layer for the classification task (see Table 6).

**Table 6.** Architecture of the RNN. 'None' indicates the batch size (set to 256).

| Layer | Output shape | # Parameters |
|---|---|---|
| LSTM | (None, 64) | 25'088 |
| Batch normalization | (None, 64) | 256 |
| Dense (sigmoid) | (None, 1) | 65 |
| Total parameters: 25'409 | Trainable parameters: 25'281 | Non-trainable parameters: 128 |

The CRNN consists of a single layer of the same RNN preceded by 3 convolutional layers (see Table 7). All the methods use the same set features, however with different window strategies.

**Table 7.** Architecture of the CRNN. 'None' indicates the batch size (set to 256).

| Layer | Output shape | # Parameters |
|---|---|---|
| 1D convolution | (None, 10, 8) | 4608 |
| Batch normalization | (None, 10, 8) | 32 |
| ReLU | (None, 10, 8) | 0 |
| Max pooling | (None, 5, 8) | 0 |
| 1D convolution | (None, 5, 16) | 1536 |
| Batch normalization | (None, 5, 16) | 64 |
| ReLU | (None, 5, 16) | 0 |
| Max pooling | (None, 2, 16) | 0 |
| 1D convolution | (None, 2, 32) | 3072 |
| Batch normalization | (None, 2, 32) | 128 |
| ReLU | (None, 2, 32) | 0 |
| Max pooling | (None, 1, 32) | 0 |
| LSTM | (None, 64) | 24'832 |
| Dense | (None, 256) | 16'640 |
| Batch normalization | (None, 256) | 1024 |
| Activation | (None, 256) | 0 |
| Dense | (None, 32) | 8224 |
| Batch normalization | (None, 32) | 128 |
| Activation | (None, 32) | 0 |
| Dense | (None, 1) | 33 |
| Total parameters: 60'321 | Trainable parameters: 59'633 | Non-trainable parameters: 688 |

**Experimental Results.** The overall results comparing the three different approaches are presented in Table 8. The performance of the best classifier is presented in Fig. 4. The threshold of the classifiers is selected according to the Youden's J statistic.

Furthermore, the impact of the phasic and tonic parts of the EDA signal is investigated by their ablation (Table 9). That is the best model is trained and tested without the presence of their related features.

**Table 8.** Evaluation of the different machine learning models and pre-processing parameters

| | Gradient boosting DT | | | | RNN | | | | CRNN | | | |
|---|---|---|---|---|---|---|---|---|---|---|---|---|
| window size [sec] | 30 | 60 | 120 | 180 | 30 | 60 | 120 | 180 | 30 | 60 | 120 | 180 |
| step size [sec] 15 | 15 | 15 | 15 | 15 | 15 | 15 | 15 | 15 | 15 | 15 | 15 | 15 |
| total # of windows | 889 | 878 | 854 | 830 | 889 | 878 | 854 | 830 | 889 | 878 | 854 | 830 |
| postive classes [%] | 43 | 43 | 44 | 46 | 43 | 43 | 44 | 46 | 43 | 43 | 44 | 46 |
| # time steps | N/A | N/A | N/A | N/A | 10 | 10 | 10 | 10 | 10 | 10 | 10 | 10 |
| AUC | 0.63 | 0.62 | 0.61 | 0.62 | 0.64 | 0.65 | 0.71 | 0.73 | 0.62 | 0.63 | 0.59 | 0.61 |
| weighted $F_1$ | 0.57 | 0.58 | 0.56 | 0.58 | 0.65 | 0.61 | 0.72 | 0.77 | 0.67 | 0.69 | 0.65 | 0.68 |
| **macro $F_1$** | 0.58 | 0.58 | 0.55 | 0.58 | 0.62 | 0.58 | **0.67** | **0.71** | **0.63** | **0.65** | 0.60 | 0.63 |
| 3-fold std macro $F_1$ | 0.08 | 0.04 | 0.05 | 0.04 | 0.02 | 0.04 | 0.06 | 0.05 | 0.05 | 0.02 | 0.04 | 0.07 |
| | Random baseline macro $F_1$: 0.48 | | | | | | | | | | | |

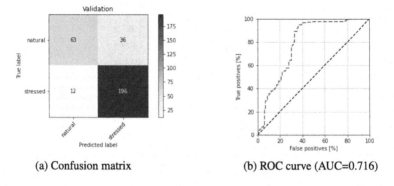

(a) Confusion matrix                           (b) ROC curve (AUC=0.716)

**Fig. 4.** Classification metrics of the best RNN model

**Table 9.** Ablation results for the EDA signal with the RNN model of the best macro $F_1$

| | All features except tonic EDA | All features except phasic EDA | All features |
|---|---|---|---|
| AUC | 0.65 | 0.71 | 0.73 |
| weighted $F_1$ | 0.67 | 0.75 | 0.77 |
| **macro $F_1$** | 0.62 | 0.68 | 0.71 |
| difference | −13% | −5% | |

## 5    Discussion

The best model for the binary classification of stress is achieved with a recurrent neural network, and yields a macro $F_1$ of 71%. In our tests, the lowest score is of 55% (because of the imbalanced nature of the dataset, the random baseline is of 48%). The AUC of the ROC curve of the best model is of 0.716, meaning that if the focus were to detect stress with a better recall, an accuracy of almost

100% could be achieved, traded off by almost 50% of false positives). We did not include other metrics (such as accuracy) because of the imbalanced nature of our dataset.

In almost every situation, RNN and CRNN outperforms decision trees. This result confirms the general idea that time series are better handled by deep learning architectures and more precisely recurrent or convolutional networks, thanks to their capacity to handle sequences of time. However, the hyper-parameters for building the time sequences may highly impact the score (from 0.58 to 0.71 in the same RNN). We were unfortunately not able to acquire more data at this stage of the project, since experimental part was planned for the beginning of March 2020, when global confinement due to COVID-19 has started. Nevertheless, even though we had only six participants, for each of them we have recorded signals, time-series, of about 35 minutes long. The feature extraction algorithms processed these time-series with window size of 1 min and step of half a minutes, thus providing a time-series of training point of 70 for each of six participants. Despite the small size of our training set, the received results are promising, especially considering a deep learning architecture.

As mentioned in Sect. 4, EDA contains information not only related to slow changes, that is the tonic component, but also in the rapid or phasic changes of the signal. We observed that the prediction of stress is strongly based rather on the tonic component, with a drop of 13% on the $F_1$ score with its ablation.

As future work, globally, we aim at developing a wearable system allowing for seamless monitoring and detection of critical signatures of stress leading to distress. To achieve this goal we still have a long road. First of all, to improve the quality of stress prediction, we intend to continue our project towards implementing a more personalized prediction, since the values contained in physiological signals are specific for each participant. For example, as was already mentioned, the value of SCL can vary widely, typically between 2–20 µS. Therefore, such factors as physical constitution as well as the baseline level of stress of participant must be taken into account. Further, we would like to take into account the ACC signal and provides a five-class definition of stress, differentiating between emotional, intellectual, and physical stress, as well as pain, in contrast to the non-stress conditions.

Once we will go from laboratory setting to everyday life our dataset will include the contextual data, as well as measurement of cortisol. Measurements of cortisol are quite intrusive. However, since some studies have presented already that slow arousal of the morning cortisol level serves as the indication of "burnout" state [13], its measurement performed with participants of the long experiments will allows us defining the signature of stress events leading to the 'burnout' or distress state. Finally, other machine learning algorithms can be implemented allowing to choose the best ones among them, in order to improve stress detection and monitoring.

# 6  Conclusion

Stress causes biochemical, physiological and behavioral changes, and can be described as an uncomfortable emotion. The long-term exposure to stress can cause illness. In this paper we have implemented a prediction stress detection system from a wrist-device sensor providing stress relevant physiological signals. We have implemented three classification algorithms providing two-class classification Stress vs Non-Stress. A reasonable prediction can be observed when we apply a recurrent neural network, this model yiels a macro $F_1$ of 71%. Our work will not stop here, and as described in Sect. 5 we have several perspectives to improve the system.

# References

1. La commission cantonale (VD) d'éthique de la recherche sur l'être humain. http://cer-vd.ch/
2. Barreto, A., Zhai, J., Adjouadi, M.: Non-intrusive physiological monitoring for automated stress detection in human-computer interaction. In: Lew, M., Sebe, N., Huang, T.S., Bakker, E.M. (eds.) HCI 2007. LNCS, vol. 4796, pp. 29–38. Springer, Heidelberg (2007). https://doi.org/10.1007/978-3-540-75773-3_4
3. Bogomolov, A., Lepri, B., Ferron, M., Pianesi, F., Pentland, A.: Daily stress recognition from mobile phone data, weather conditions and individual traits. In: Proceedings of the 22nd ACM International Conference on Multimedia, pp. 477–486 (2014)
4. Boucsein, W.: Electrodermal indices of emotion and stress. In: Electrodermal Activity, pp. 369–391 (1992). Chapter 3
5. Boucsein, W., et al.: Society for psychophysiological research ad hoc committee on electrodermal measures. Publication recommendations for electrodermal measurements. Psychophysiology 49(8), 1017–1034 (2012)
6. Ciabattoni, L., Ferracuti, F., Longhi, S., Pepa, L., Romeo, L., Verdini, F.: Real-time mental stress detection based on smartwatch. In: 2017 IEEE International Conference on Consumer Electronics (ICCE), pp. 110–111. IEEE (2017)
7. Doberenz, S., Roth, W.T., Wollburg, E., Maslowski, N.I., Kim, S.: Methodological considerations in ambulatory skin conductance monitoring. Int. J. Psychophysiol. 80(2), 87–95 (2011)
8. Han, H., Byun, K., Kang, H.G.: A deep learning-based stress detection algorithm with speech signal. In: Proceedings of the 2018 Workshop on Audio-Visual Scene Understanding for Immersive Multimedia, pp. 11–15 (2018)
9. Hernando, A., et al.: Inclusion of respiratory frequency information in heart rate variability analysis for stress assessment. IEEE J. Biomed. Health Inform. 20(4), 1016–1025 (2016)
10. Kurniawan, H., Maslov, A.V., Pechenizkiy, M.: Stress detection from speech and galvanic skin response signals. In: Proceedings of the 26th IEEE International Symposium on Computer-Based Medical Systems, pp. 209–214. IEEE (2013)
11. Liao, C.Y., Chen, R.C., Tai, S.K.: Emotion stress detection using EEG signal and deep learning technologies. In: 2018 IEEE International Conference on Applied System Invention (ICASI), pp. 90–93. IEEE (2018)

12. LiKamWa, R., Liu, Y., Lane, N.D., Zhong, L.: MoodScope: building a mood sensor from smartphone usage patterns. In: Proceeding of the 11th Annual International Conference on Mobile Systems, Applications, and Services, pp. 389–402 (2013)
13. Marchand, A., Juster, R.P., Durand, P., Lupien, S.J.: Burnout symptom sub-types and cortisol profiles: what's burning most? Psychoneuroendocrinology **40**, 27–36 (2014)
14. Posada-Quintero, H.F., Florian, J.P., Orjuela-Cañón, A.D., Chon, K.H.: Electro-dermal activity is sensitive to cognitive stress under water. Front. Physiol. **8**, 1128 (2018)
15. Salahuddin, L., Jeong, M.G., Kim, D., Lim, S.K., Won, K., Woo, J.M.: Dependence of heart rate variability on stress factors of stress response inventory. In: 2007 9th International Conference on e-Health Networking, Application and Services, pp. 236–239. IEEE (2007)
16. Sano, A., Picard, R.W.: Stress recognition using wearable sensors and mobile phones. In: 2013 Humaine Association Conference on Affective Computing and Intelligent Interaction, pp. 671–676. IEEE (2013)
17. Schmidt, P., Reiss, A., Duerichen, R., Marberger, C., Van Laerhoven, K.: Intro-ducing WESAD, a multimodal dataset for wearable stress and affect detection. In: Proceedings of the 20th ACM International Conference on Multimodal Interaction, pp. 400–408 (2018)
18. Schneiderman, N., Ironson, G., Siegel, S.D.: Stress and health: psychological, behavioral, and biological determinants. Annu. Rev. Clin. Psychol. **1**, 607–628 (2005)
19. Shukla, J., Barreda-Angeles, M., Oliver, J., Nandi, G., Puig, D.: Feature extraction and selection for emotion recognition from electrodermal activity. IEEE Trans. Affect. Comput. (2019)
20. Stalder, T., et al.: Assessment of the cortisol awakening response: expert consensus guidelines. Psychoneuroendocrinology **63**, 414–432 (2016)
21. Zubair, M., Yoon, C., Kim, H., Kim, J., Kim, J.: Smart wearable band for stress detection. In: 2015 5th International Conference on IT Convergence and Security (ICITCS), pp. 1–4. IEEE (2015)

# Classification of Anxiety Based on EDA and HR

Raquel Sebastião[(⊠)][iD]

Institute of Electronics and Informatics Engineering of Aveiro (IEETA),
Department of Electronics, Telecommunications and Informatics (DETI),
University of Aveiro, 3810-193 Aveiro, Portugal
`raquel.sebastiao@ua.pt`

**Abstract.** This work presents anxiety classification using physiological data, namely, EDA (eletrodermal activity) and HR (heart rate), collected with a sensing wrist-wearable device during a neutral baseline state condition. For this purpose, the WESAD public available dataset was used. The baseline condition was collected for around 20 min on 15 participants. Afterwards, to assess anxiety scores, the shortened 6-item STAI was filled by the participants. Using train and test sets with 70% and 30% of data, respectively, the proposed ensemble of 100 bagged classification trees obtained an overall accuracy of 95.7%. This, along with the high precision and recall obtained, reveal the good performance of the proposed classifier and support the ability of anxiety score classification using physiological data. Such a classification task can be integrated in a mobile application presenting coping strategies to deal and manage anxiety.

**Keywords:** Anxiety · Physiological data · Heart rate · Eletrodermal activity · Wearable measurements · Mobile applications

## 1 Introduction

Considering that it is of utmost importance to properly assess anxiety, recent studies stress out alterations of physiological signals related with it. Occasional anxiety, which is expected to be experienced along lifetime, is related with temporary worry or fear when facing a particular situation. Anxiety disorders go beyond temporary. In those cases, anxiety occurs frequently and at undue time,

The author acknowledge the public availability of WESAD dataset. This work was supported by the Portuguese Science Foundation (FCT) through national funds, within IEETA/UA R&D unit (UIDB/00127/2020). This work is also funded by national funds, European Regional Development Fund, FSE through COMPETE2020, through FCT, in the scope of the framework contract foreseen in the numbers 4, 5, and 6 of the article 23, of the Decree-Law 57/2016, of August 29, changed by Law 57/2017, of July 19. Moreover, this work is funded by national funds through FCT – Fundação para a Ciência e a Tecnologia, I.P., under the Scientific Employment Stimulus - Individual Call - CEECIND/03986/2018.

© ICST Institute for Computer Sciences, Social Informatics and Telecommunications Engineering 2021
Published by Springer Nature Switzerland AG 2021. All Rights Reserved
R. Goleva et al. (Eds.): HealthyIoT 2020, LNICST 360, pp. 112–123, 2021.
https://doi.org/10.1007/978-3-030-69963-5_8

it does not go way and get worse over time [3]. When diagnosed, the treatment can rely on medication, on behavioural therapy or on the combination of both.

In 2019, anxiety disorders were estimated to affect 4.05% of the world population, mostly women [2], with serious implications in quality of life, daily activities, workplace, families and society [20]. Anxiety disorders are affecting 301 million people, cutting across age groups, and with an increasing trend. This growing estimate are of major concern, and coping strategies to deal with anxiety disorders are of great interest. In Portugal, it affects 9.08% of the population [2], a percentage of great relevance when comparing with worldwide data.

Regarding the global rise of the consumption of antidepressants, according to the OECD (Organisation for Economic Co-operation and Development) indicators [1], in 2017, Portugal was the fifth country of the OECD with the highest consumption of antidepressants, with 104 daily doses per thousand people. Although it may be associated with a greater recognition and diagnosis of anxiety and depression disorders, it clearly reveals the increase of incidence of these disorders when compared to 2000 (when the consumption was estimated to be slightly below one third).

Considering this rise, awareness and attention need to be devoted to mental illness, and strategies to deal and manage anxiety are crucially needed. More than ever, due to COVID-19 pandemic, and considering the disrupt situation that we are facing and social distancing, anxiety can become overwhelming.

## 1.1   Motivation, Goals and Outline

The rational above, reinforces the urge of cognitive-behavioural therapies, accessible at a glance, helping people with anxiety disorders, presenting different ways of thinking, behaving, and reacting to anxiety-producing and fearful objects and situations [3].

Sensing wrist-wearable devices grant the easy and on the fly measurement of physiological signals, which can be integrated with a mobile application (app) for anxiety classification based on these physiological signals. Therefore, such a classification system can be integrated within a mobile app for self-management strategies to deal, in real time, with anxiety symptoms.

In a university context, this app could have significant improvements in students' well-being, helping to overcome daily and recurrent stressful situations, such as works' or projects' deadlines, exams, oral presentations, among others.

Targeting the psychophysiological perspective of anxiety, this work aims to provide motivation and support for the development of a mobile app with coping strategies to deal with anxiety, based on the ecological momentary assessment of the anxiety of the users through the analysis of EDA and HR.

Therefore, the goal of this study is to classify anxiety through physiological signals from data without any affective state elicitation. Thus, using data gathered with a Empatica wristband [7], this work presents anxiety classification, based on EDA and HR collected during a baseline neutral state condition.

The obtained results allow the identification of physiological correlates of anxiety states and can be further integrated into wearable and smart sensing contexts. Indeed, the results support the feasibility and encourage the development of a mobile app, that connected with a similar wristband, and according to anxiety score classification, can present coping strategies to deal and manage with it.

For these purposes, it was used the WESAD multimodal dataset [18], containing self-reports, motion and physiological data, recorded with a wristband (Empatica wristband) and a chest-worn device (Biosignalsplux RespiBAN Professional), of 15 participants during a lab study designed for stress and affect detection.

The remain of this work is organized as follow. Section 2 presents related works on anxiety disorders and mobile applications to deal with it. Section 3, after a brief description of the dataset used, presents the methodology used. Afterwards, Sect. 4 compares and discusses the results on relating EDA and HR with anxiety and on anxiety classification. Concluding remarks and possibilities for further research are presented in Sect. 5.

## 2    Related Works

In the past decade, several studies have shown that common symptoms associated with anxiety are alterations in HRV (heart rate variability), HR and sweating [6,9,10,12,13,17,18]. However, the physiological relation with anxiety is still an open problem. These findings may open new doors to cognitive behavioural therapies helping control and manage anxiety, particularly given the accessibility and affordability of new wearable technologies, such as wristbands, allowing the continuous collection of physiological data.

Moreover, these biomedical sensors are often wireless and can stream to several and small devices, like smartphones, supporting the feasibility of the analysis of physiological signals and assisting with suggestions to deal with anxiety. Indeed, more recently, due to the increasing concern on mental disorders, namely anxiety, and to the technological advances which widespread the access and usage of mobile devices, there had been proposed mobile applications to help users dealing with anxiety [4,16,19,21].

The work [8] provides a review on e-health treatments for anxiety, showing the efficacy of internet-delivered cognitive behavioural therapies to deal with anxiety disorders and identifying the limitations in engaging patients. Moreover, the authors also addressed the potential of mobile apps and virtual reality interventions for the treatment of anxiety symptoms, supporting their feasibility.

More recently, [19] provides a review supporting the use of mobile apps as helpful and accessible tools in the assessment and treatment of anxiety in youth. Although, the overall good results concerning ease of use and acceptability, and high satisfaction ratings, the authors pointed out the burdensome of user engagement over time, as well the work [8].

Regarding applications for self-management of symptoms related to mental disorders, the work [4] proposed the use of the Mindfulness Meditation app, showing the relevance of embracing HRV in the assessment and treatment of these conditions, and providing a step further in the feasibility of using HRV as a biomarker and biofeedback tool within clinical and health psychology.

Although not addressing physiological responses, the work [16] contributes with an evaluation of the effectiveness of the Feel Stress Free app, useful for the treatment of depression and anxiety symptoms. During a 6-week trial with 168 university students, this cognitive behavioural therapy-based app, which provides relaxation activities, mood tracking and thought challenging, and minigames, shown promising results to deal with depression and anxiety symptoms.

On the other hand, the work [13] proposes the assessment of mental well-being and health through a mobile application for HRV analysis, showing a positive relationship between both.

The authors of the used dataset (WESAD) provided a study on classifying different affective states (neutral, stress, amusement), using a protocol specifically designed for elicitation of the affective states [18]. Besides comparing the chest and wrist devices, in this threeclass classification problem (baseline vs. stress vs. amusement), the authors reached accuracies up to 93%.

Depart from studies relying on the elicitation of affective states, the presented work relies only on data collected during the baseline, representing a neutral state condition without any elicitation.

## 3   Data and Methodology

This section briefly describes the WESAD dataset, explaining the physiological signals used for the purpose of anxiety classification, the methodology to achieve them and the evaluation metrics to assess the obtained results. All the data pre-processing and processing and statistical evaluations were performed using MATLAB R2019b [15].

### 3.1   WESAD Dataset and Physiological Data Used

WESAD is a public available multimodal dataset[1], containing self-reports, motion and physiological data of 15 participants during a lab study designed for stress and affect detection, recorded with the Empatica wristband [7] (namely, blood volume pulse - BVP, electrodermal activity, body temperature and three-axis acceleration), and with the Biosignalsplux RespiBAN Professional chest-worn device [5] (namely, electrocardiogram, electrodermal activity, electromyogram, respiration, body temperature and three-axis acceleration). The authors also provide the average heart rate extracted from the BVP signal. According to the goals, the protocol for collecting WESAD dataset was designed with several conditions in two different combinations.

---

[1] https://archive.ics.uci.edu/ml/datasets/WESAD+%28Wearable+Stress+and+Affect+Detection\%29\#.

To attain the purpose of anxiety classification, this study used only the data collected during the baseline condition, which aimed to reflect a neutral affective state while participants were sitting/standing at a table with neutral reading material. For class identification, as ground truth, it was used the responses of participants, after baseline condition, to the shortened 6-item STAI (Spielberger State-Trait Anxiety Inventory), varying from a minimum score of 4 to a maximum score of 24, which offers a briefer and acceptable scale, while remains sensitive to different degrees of anxiety [14]. In the 6-item STAI, participant scored from "1" = "Not at all" to "4" = "Very much so", the following 6 conditions:

- I feel at ease
- I feel nervous
- I am jittery
- I am relaxed
- I am worried
- I feel pleasant

As the goal of this study is to classify the self-reported anxiety through physiological signals, it relies on data without any affective state elicitation, therefore data collected during a baseline condition ($mean$ = 19.57 min and $std$ = 0.26 min), and the results from the 6-item STAI (with summed scores ranged from 10 to 16). Figure 1 shows the EDA and HR signals for participants with minimum and maximum, respectively, upper and bottom, anxiety scores in the 6-item STAI. For these participants, from the HR signals, it can not be stressed out any pattern or trend. However, it can be observed considerable differences regarding the EDA signal, which is significantly higher for a great STAI score.

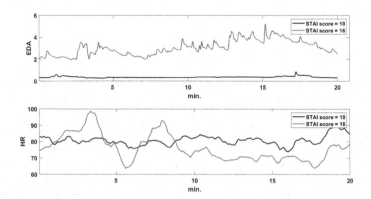

**Fig. 1.** EDA and HR (upper and bottom, respectively) of two participants with STAI score of 10 and 16 (minimum and maximum in this dataset).

## 3.2   Methodology for Anxiety Classification

Aiming at classify anxiety through physiological signals, the first step concerns the categorization of participants according to anxiety scores, which in this dataset ranges from 10 to 16, distributed according to the Fig. 2. As it can be observed, the majority class corresponds to a score of 12 in the 6-item STAI, while scores of 15 and 16, are the minority classes. Although data is not equally distributed, this work will not use any technique to deal with imbalanced datasets. Instead, it relies on other evaluation metrics, rather than only accuracy, to assess the performance of the classifier.

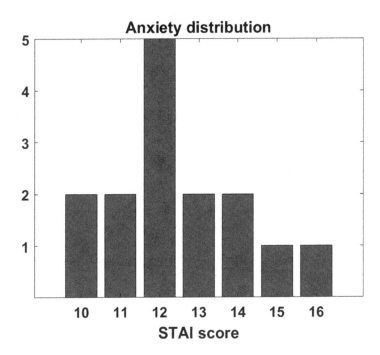

**Fig. 2.** Anxiety distribution, according to the score in the 6-item STAI, of WESAD dataset participants.

Regarding the EDA, collected at a sample rate of 4 Hz, and the HR, computed from the BVP, the box plots of both were analysed to explore the differences between the EDA and HR medians of different STAI scores, for all participants, during the baseline condition.

To analyse the differences between STAI scores, it was first applied the Lilliefors test to decide if data comes from a normal distributed family. Both EDA and HR failed to be normal distributed.

Therefore, to perform a global evaluation, was applied the Kruskal-Wallis (KW) Test [11], a nonparametric test, that allows to decide if the samples from the different STAI scores were originated from the same distribution, by comparing the mean ranks of EDA and HR of the different scores.

In case of differences between the score groups, those are further analysed, through multiple comparisons between the groups. In this case, is used the multcompare function from MATLAB, which besides returning the pairwise comparison results based on the KS outputs, also allows an interactive graphical multiple comparison of the groups, displaying the rank mean estimates and the comparison intervals for each group.

To decide on the best method for classifying anxiety scores through EDA and HR measured during the baseline condition, it was created an ensemble of learners for classification with data from the 15 participants, using bagging, adaptive boosting and random undersampling boosting (to deal with the imbalance of the dataset) algorithms.

Afterwards, using the best method to fit the ensemble with the EDA and HR data to STAI scores, data from baseline was used to estimate the misclassification rate and confusion matrix using 5-fold cross-validation.

Finally, this ensemble was trained with 70% of EDA and HR data, and the remain 30% of the data, held out for testing, was used on the model to make predictions.

### 3.3   Evaluation Metrics

The accuracy of a model is not a recommended measure to use in class imbalanced problems, as it translates performance of a model by dividing the number of corrected classifications by the total number of data examples.

Therefore, to evaluate the performance of the classifier, the confusion matrix was calculated, allowing to compute quality metrics as *Precision* and *Recall*. The *Precision* gives the ratio between the correct predictions (TP) and all the predictions of a given class, true positives plus false positives (TP+FP), and the *Recall* is defined as the ratio between the examples of a class that were correctly classified on this class, true positives plus false negatives (TP+FN). For both, the closer to 100%, the better the results are. Indeed, in the case of both get high values, then classes are properly handled by the classifier.

Combining both, the $F_1$ measure is the harmonic mean of *Precision* and *Recall*.

$$Precision = \frac{TP}{TP + FP}, Recall = \frac{TP}{TP + FN} \text{ and } F_1 = 2\frac{Precision * Recall}{Precision + Recall}$$

## 4   Results

Regarding the distribution of EDA and HR values of the 15 participants, Fig. 3 show the box plots of EDA and HR for the 15 participants under study. The left and right figures show the EDA and HR, respectively, according to anxiety scores from the 6-item STAI. The left figure points out, with 95% confidence, that the

EDA medians of the STAI scores 11, 12 and 16 are different, as the notches in the box plots do not overlap. With respect to the right figure, it shows, with 95% confidence, that the HR medians of the STAI scores 10, 11, 12, 14 and 15 are different. Therefore, using both as features to predict anxiety score would be an advantage, as one surpasses the drawbacks of the other.

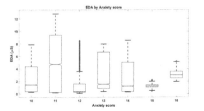 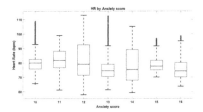

**Fig. 3.** Box plots of EDA and HR (left and right, respectively) for the 15 participants in WESAD dataset.

An analysis of the box plots, allows to observe the EDA and HR differences between the different anxiety scores. The EDA associated with anxiety scores 11, 13 and 14 present a higher variability, while EDA from anxiety scores 15 and 16 present smaller variability. When anxiety scored 12, EDA presented a great number of outlier values. Regarding HR, for anxiety scores of 10, 13 and 15, it can be observed a great number of outliers, while when anxiety scored 12 and 14, despite without outliers, the HR presented a higher variability.

With respect to the Kruskal-Wallis test performed using the EDA and HR data of the 15 participants, the returned p-value ($0 < 0.01$, for both cases) indicates that, at a significance level of 1%, the null hypothesis that the EDA, or HR, from the different anxiety scores (6-item STAI) come from the same distribution is rejected.

As the Kruskal-Wallis test allowed to conclude that the median values of EDA and HR from the different anxiety scores are significant different, it is performed multiple comparisons tests to reveal which from the 7 groups are significant different from the others.

Figure 4 presents the estimates of the mean rank order of EDA and HR values, and 99% confidence comparison intervals, for the anxiety scores. Regarding EDA (left), it can be concluded that groups with anxiety score of 12 and 14 have mean ranks significantly different from all the remain 6 scores, while anxiety scores 10, 11 and 15 only presented mean ranks significantly different from scores 12, 13, 14 and 16, and scores 13 and 16 have mean ranks not significantly different from each other. With respect to HR (right), with the exception of anxiety scores 10 and 15 and anxiety scores 13 and 16, that present mean ranks not significantly different from each other, the remain anxiety scores (11, 12 and 14) have mean ranks significantly different from all the remain 6 scores.

The presented analysis, concludes with the construction of a classifier, using these time series (EDA and HR) as features, to predict the different anxiety scores during the baseline condition.

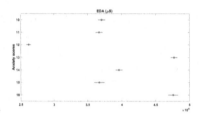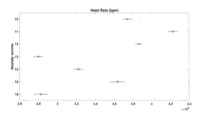

**Fig. 4.** Multicomparison graphics for the mean rank of EDA and HR (left and right, respectively) grouped by the 7 anxiety scores (6-item STAI).

At first, to decide on the best method for classifying anxiety scores, it was constructed a predictive classification ensemble using all available predictor variables in EDA and HR data (71684 samples, corresponding to around 20 min of baseline condition from 15 participants, collected at a sample rate of 4 Hz). After optimization, results suggested that the best method was bagging, with random predictor selections at each split (random forest).

Therefore, using all the available data, the misclassification rate and confusion matrix were estimated, using 5-fold cross-validation, obtaining an estimate cross-validated classification error of 3.77%. The obtained confusion matrix, presented in Table 1, shows, for all the classes, high values of true positives (correct predictions), displayed in the principal diagonal of the matrix, and small values (when compared to these) of true negatives, false positives and false negatives.

**Table 1.** Confusion matrix of anxiety classification using EDA and HR during the baseline condition.

|  |  | Predicted anxiety score | | | | | | |
|---|---|---|---|---|---|---|---|---|
|  |  | 10 | 11 | 12 | 13 | 14 | 15 | 16 |
|  | 10 | 9092 | 55 | 103 | 141 | 134 | 36 | 39 |
|  | 11 | 65 | 9313 | 123 | 46 | 38 | 3 | 0 |
|  | 12 | 124 | 123 | 23295 | 82 | 109 | 158 | 29 |
| Anxiety score STAI | 13 | 54 | 21 | 82 | 9391 | 67 | 41 | 0 |
|  | 14 | 149 | 28 | 104 | 113 | 8977 | 20 | 113 |
|  | 15 | 28 | 4 | 161 | 40 | 16 | 4358 | 9 |
|  | 16 | 99 | 0 | 25 | 0 | 116 | 1 | 4559 |

Finally, due to the good results obtained so far, an ensemble of 100 bagged classification trees was trained using 70% of the data (50179 samples). The remain 30% of data were used to test the ensemble (21505 samples). Both test and train sets were constructed preserving the original class distribution.

The obtained accuracy of 95.7% is reinforced by the obtained high values for the precision, recall and $F_1$, which indicate a good performance of the classifier, validating its capability to classify anxiety scores using EDA and HR data. For each of anxiety scores, or classes, the precision, recall and $F_1$ are presented at Table 2.

**Table 2.** Precision, recall and $F_1$ measure for classifying anxiety scores using EDA and HR during the baseline condition.

| Anxiety score | Precision | Recall | $F_1$ score |
|---|---|---|---|
| 10 | 96.953 | 96.656 | 96.804 |
| 11 | 97.47 | 96.453 | 96.959 |
| 12 | 93.951 | 95.451 | 94.695 |
| 13 | 92.482 | 94.152 | 93.309 |
| 14 | 93.564 | 93.827 | 93.695 |
| 15 | 96.641 | 96.341 | 96.491 |
| 16 | 95.077 | 93.889 | 94.479 |

## 5  Conclusions and Further Research

The recent global increase of anxiety disorders and the rise of the consumption of antidepressants, demands that awareness and attention need to be devoted to mental illness. Therefore, coping strategies to deal and manage with anxiety are crucially. Moreover, sensing wrist-wearable devices, which are a minimally invasive equipment that can assess, continuously and with low-compliance, physiological signals, offers an excellent opportunity to monitor the physiological alterations under different conditions, namely stress and anxiety.

In this context, this work targets the psychophysiological perspective of anxiety, providing motivation and support for the development of a mobile app with coping strategies to deal with anxiety, based on the ecological momentary assessment of the anxiety of the users through the analysis of EDA and HR.

It proposes an ensemble of 100 bagged classification trees that, presenting an overall accuracy of 95.7% and precision, recall and $F_1$ means, for all classes, of 95.16%, 95.25% and 95.20%, respectively, shows to be feasible to classify anxiety scores through EDA and HR collected with Empatica, a wrist-wearable device. These results allow the identification of physiological correlates of anxiety states and can be further integrated into wearable and smart sensing contexts.

Although relying in a public available dataset with 15 participants, the encouraging obtained results sustain a future design of a protocol specially fitted to this problem.

Moreover, further research will devote efforts to develop a mobile app, that receiving physiological data collected with a wearable wrist device, classifies anxiety states and provides feedback and strategies to deal with anxiety.

# References

1. Health at a glance 2019: OECD indicators (2019). https://doi.org/10.1787/4dd50c09-en. Accessed 16 Nov 2020
2. GBD results tool, global health data exchange (GHDx). http://ghdx.healthdata.org/gbd-results-tool. Accessed 21 Aug 2020
3. Anxiety disorders, the National Institute of Mental Health (NIMH). https://www.nimh.nih.gov/index.shtml. Accessed 16 Nov 2020
4. Azam, M.A., Latman, V.V., Katz, J.: Effects of a 12-min smartphone-based mindful breathing task on heart rate variability for students with clinically relevant chronic pain, depression, and anxiety: protocol for a randomized controlled trial. JMIR Res. Protoc. **8**(12), e14119 (2019). https://doi.org/10.2196/14119
5. Biosignalsplux: respiban professional. https://biosignalsplux.com/products/wearables/respiban-pro.html. Accessed 22 Aug 2020
6. Blom, E.H., Olsson, E., Serlachius, E., Ericson, M., Ingvar, M.: Heart rate variability (HRV) in adolescent females with anxiety disorders and major depressive disorder. Acta Paediatrica **99**(4), 604–611 (2010). https://doi.org/10.1111/j.1651-2227.2009.01657.x
7. Empatica: E4 wristband. https://www.empatica.com/en-eu/research/e4/, Accessed 22 Aug 2020
8. Firth, J., Torous, J., Carney, R., Newby, J., Cosco, T.D., Christensen, H., Sarris, J.: Digital technologies in the treatment of anxiety: Recent innovations and future directions. Curr. Psychiatry Rep. **20**(6) (2018). https://doi.org/10.1007/s11920-018-0910-2
9. Huang, H., Wan, K.: Heart rate variability in junior high school students with depression and anxiety in Taiwan. Acta Neuropsychiatrica **25**(3), 175–178 (2013). https://doi.org/10.1111/acn.12010
10. van der Kooy, K.G., van Hout, H.P., van Marwijk, H.W., de Haan, M., Stehouwer, C., Beekman, A.T.: Differences in heart rate variability between depressed and non-depressed elderly. Int. J. Geriatr. Psychiatry **21**(2), 147–150 (2006). https://doi.org/10.1002/gps.1439
11. Kruskal, W.H., Wallis, W.A.: Use of ranks in one-criterion variance analysis. J. Am. Stat. Assoc. **47**(260), 583–621 (1952). https://doi.org/10.1080/01621459.1952.10483441
12. Licht, C., de Geus, E.J.C., van Dyck, R., Penninx, B.W.J.H.: Association between anxiety disorders and heart rate variability in the Netherlands study of depression and anxiety (NESDA). Psychosomatic Med. **71**(5), 508–518 (2009). https://doi.org/10.1097/PSY.0b013e3181a292a6
13. Liu, I., Ni, S., Peng, K.: Happiness at your fingertips: assessing mental health with smartphone photoplethysmogram-based heart rate variability analysis. Telemedicine and e-Health published online ahead of print (2020). https://doi.org/10.1089/tmj.2019.0283, pMID: 32101084
14. Marteau, T.M., Bekker, H.: The development of a six-item short-form of the state scale of the spielberger statetrait anxiety inventory (stai). Br. J. Clin. Psychol. **31**(3), 301–306 (1992). https://doi.org/10.1111/j.2044-8260.1992.tb00997.x
15. MATLAB: R2019b. The MathWorks Inc., Natick, Massachusetts (2019)
16. McCloud, T., Jones, R., Lewis, G., Bell, V., Tsakanikos, E.: Effectiveness of a mobile app intervention for anxiety and depression symptoms in university students: randomized controlled trial. JMIR Mhealth Uhealth **8**(7), e15418 (2020). https://doi.org/10.2196/15418

17. Nikolic, M., Aktar, E., Bagels, S., Colonnesi, C., de Vente, W.: Bumping heart and sweaty palms: physiological hyperarousal as a risk factor for child social anxiety. J. Child Psychol. Psychiatry **59**(2), 119–128 (2018). https://doi.org/10.1111/jcpp. 12813

18. Schmidt, P., Reiss, A., Duerichen, R., Marberger, C., Van Laerhoven, K.: Introducing wesad, a multimodal dataset for wearable stress and affect detection. In: Proceedings of the 20th ACM International Conference on Multimodal Interaction, pp. 400–408. ICMI 2018, Association for Computing Machinery, New York (2018). https://doi.org/10.1145/3242969.3242985

19. Temkin, A.B., Schild, J., Falk, A., Bennett, S.M.: Mobile apps for youth anxiety disorders: a review of the evidence and forecast of future innovations. Prof. Psychol.: Res. Pract. **51**(4), 400–413 (2020). https://doi.org/10.1037/pro0000342

20. W.H.O.: Mental health (WHO). https://www.who.int/mentalhealth/ intheworkplace/en/. Accessed 21 Aug 2020

21. Yin, H., et al.: Mobile mental health apps in China: systematic app store search. J. Med. Internet Res. **22**(7), e14915 (2020). https://doi.org/10.2196/14915

# Preliminary Results of IoT-Enabled EDA-Based Analysis of Physiological Response to Acoustic Stimuli

Angelica Poli[ID], Anna Brocanelli, Stefania Cecchi[ID], Simone Orcioni[ID],
and Susanna Spinsante[(✉)][ID]

Department of Information Engineering, Università Politecnica delle Marche,
60131 Ancona, Italy
{a.poli,s.cecchi,s.orcioni,s.spinsante}@staff.univpm.it,
a.brocanelli@pm.univpm.it

**Abstract.** Emotions play a key role in everyday life of human beings, and since several years, researchers have investigated the physiological changes caused by external stimuli, looking for methods to automatically classify the emotional involvement of individuals. The Galvanic Skin Response, or ElectroDermal Activity, is one of the most interesting signals used in emotion research. In this preliminary study, a few participants were submitted to auditory stimuli (i.e., pleasant, neutral and unpleasant sounds) and their skin conductance signals were measured by means of a wireless and IoT-enabled wearable device, the Empatica E4. To investigate the impact of the emotional stimuli, data measured as emotion elicitation and retrieved from the Empatica cloud platform, was analysed in the time domain, showing that pleasant and neutral sounds do not produce evident effects, while listening to an unpleasant sound increases the subjective response, with higher impact when the sound duration is shorter. The preliminary outcomes obtained confirm great intra- and inter-subject variability that deserves further investigation, by involving a bigger population of test users.

**Keywords:** ElectroDermal Activity · Galvanic Skin Response · Wearable device · Emotions · Acoustic stimuli

## 1 Introduction

In the last decades, human emotion recognition has gained growing worldwide interest in many application fields, especially healthcare [15] and neuromarketing [25]. Initially, speech analytic [16], facial expressions [7] and self-reports have

Supported by the More Years Better Lives JPI and the Italian Ministero dell'Istruzione, Università e Ricerca within the project PAAL-Privacy-Aware and Acceptable Lifelogging services for older and frail people (Grant no: PAAL JTC2017, CUP: I36G17000380001), and by Università Politecnica delle Marche with the funded research project MEMOS (RSA-B2019-DII).

© ICST Institute for Computer Sciences, Social Informatics and Telecommunications Engineering 2021
Published by Springer Nature Switzerland AG 2021. All Rights Reserved
R. Goleva et al. (Eds.): HealthyIoT 2020, LNICST 360, pp. 124–136, 2021.
https://doi.org/10.1007/978-3-030-69963-5_9

been used for human emotion detection. However, such approaches are not reliable to detect emotions, especially if the subjects under test want to hide their feelings. A reliable approach, on the other hand, may be designed around the use of physiological signals, from which objective measurements can be derived, to detect the actual emotional changes of subjects. Among physiological signals, recently the Galvanic Skin Response (GSR) has gained huge interest, thanks to the availability of wearable devices to measure it, and nowadays it is one of the most involved signals in emotion research. GSR, named also as Electrodermal Activity (EDA) or Skin Conductance (SC), is a biometric index reflecting changes in the electrical properties of the skin [23]. When humans are exposed to stimuli such as images, sounds and physical efforts, the sympathetic division of the Autonomic Nervous System (ANS), with no conscious control, induces a sweat reaction. By using two electrodes positioned on specific regions of the skin surface (e.g., fingers, hand and foot palm), the fluctuations of the skin's electrical properties can be measured [21]. The gathered information is double: the tonic component (i.e., Skin Conductance Level, SCL) related to slow changing baseline levels as individual background characteristics, and the phasic component (i.e., Skin Conductance Response, SCR) corresponding to the fast changing signal contribution which can be event-related [19].

The development of Internet of Things (IoT)-enabled wearable devices with wireless technology support has allowed and facilitated the shift from the measurement of GSR in laboratory settings, usually with bulky wired instruments, to minimally-invasive, comfortable and real-time recordings, in free-living conditions [4] with devices capable of streaming their data to a cloud-based repository.

Hereby we propose an approach to investigate whether and how the GSR signal changes in response to external stimuli, namely auditory ones, by examining the morphological characteristics of this specific physiological signal. In order to measure the impact of auditory emotional stimuli, a small dataset was collected from seven individuals both at rest condition and during the sound listening, using a single wrist-worn device with electrodes located on the bracelet. The information extracted from the GSR signals was compared against the subjects' own evaluation of their emotional status, using a standardised classification scale. After describing the methodology for the acquisition and the elaboration of the GSR signals, the results are evaluated by using statistical metrics.

The paper is organized as follows: Sect. 2 shortly reviews the state-of-the-art about GSR changes under different stimuli and the related issues. Section 3 presents the main steps of the work, including the materials and the methods to collect and process data. Section 5 presents and discusses the results obtained, including statistical metrics used. Finally, Sect. 6 concludes the paper.

## 2   Background

This section reviews the state-of-the-art about emotion investigation based on the physiological reactions.

By stimulating emotional responses with external stimuli, bodily variations (e.g., heart rate and skin conductance) can be measured. Among the most common stimuli, the video stimuli are widely delivered trying to evoke strong responses [22]. For example, Dominguez et al. [5] used 2 short video clips to elicit sadness, amusement and neutral reactions. The results show that by collecting only the GSR data, the target emotions raised can be well-recognised, especially from Random Forest (RF) classifier (up to 100% of accuracy). However, the physiological changes are highly affected by the subject's personal, cultural and cognitive aspects (e.g., expectations and perceptions) [20]. To tackle this issue, other approaches, like the work proposed by Zhao et al. [27], recorded multi-physiological signals (i.e., EDA, heart rate variability (HRV) and skin temperature), but the average accuracy of the emotion recognition process dropped down to 75.56%. It is interesting to notice how, since the native culture may affect the emotional response, data were collected by Chinese participants before and during watching Chinese video clips.

Other studies employed 2D visual stimuli selected from the International Affective Picture System (IAPS), a large database of pictures [3]. For example Dumitriu et al. [6] evaluated different emotion classification techniques, by extracting 166 images, among which pleasant and unpleasant pictures for exciting feelings, and neutral ones for calm emotions. Also in real-life scenario, Myroniv et al. [14] used images from IAPS as a triggering mechanism for the investigation of positive, neutral, and negative emotions. The proposed system included three off-the-shelf wearable biosensors (i.e., heart rate, EDA, and skin temperature sensors) to measure physiological signals, and six different Machine Learning (ML) algorithms were applied to recognise the corresponding emotional statuses. From the experiments, the proposed system achieved up to 97% recognition accuracy by adopting the k-Nearest Neighbour (k-NN) classifier.

An alternative to visual stimuli is represented by auditory stimuli. In this case, the International Affective Digital Sounds (IADS) [26] database is among the most used repositories, containing a huge collection of sound clips, together with classification labels generated by using the Self-Assessment Manikin (SAM) and three basic-emotion rating scales. However, relatively few studies have investigated the GSR response under auditory stimuli. Pozzi et al. [9], in his master thesis, aimed to understand how the relationship between music and emotion is structured. To do this, he suggested to investigate and to merge the features from both physiological and audio signals. Although the framework reached good results, some issues due to the subjective nature of emotion perception are declared (e.g., the reliability of ground truth data and the evaluation of prediction results). Such issues strongly affect the recognition accuracy, as detailed in [13] where the final percentage shifts from 95% to 70% for subject-dependent and subject-independent classification, respectively. According to Duncan et al. [24], the GSR data are also strictly influenced by the interaction between music and familiarity, which induces learned emotional responses rather than totally unconscious experiences. For this reason, other researchers such as Hu et al. [11], explored the possibility of using combinations of physiological signals (i.e., HRV and EDA) to detect users emotion response to music, considering also the personality and music preferences.

As mentioned above, whatever stimulus is used to elicit an emotion, this is supposed to affect participants' cognitive, and consequently physiological status. To combine the users' perception of an emotional stimulus together with the physiological recordings, self-assessment questionnaires have been used in literature, such as the above-mentioned SAM [2]. However, the mentioned studies are mostly focused on the emotion classification, performed by extracting features to feed and test several ML algorithms. In order to obtain a high performance from such an automatic approach to emotion detection, a detailed analysis of the GSR measurement data properties is essential. Therefore, we propose a preliminary study to investigate the characteristics of the physiological signals in response to acoustic stimuli, namely by analysing the event-related changes in GSR curve morphology. Such signals are measured in real-life contexts, i.e. out of a lab, thanks to the use of the Empatica E4 device, which may open new possibilities in terms of exploitation of physiological information generated from wearable devices.

## 3 Materials and Methods

### 3.1 Measurement Device

Data was acquired using a single wearable device, called Empatica E4[1]: a multi-sensor wristband device designed for comfortable, real-time and continuous data acquisition in everyday life. According to the datasheet provided by the manufacturer [8], four sensors are embedded in such a device, namely a photoplethysmographic sensor (PPG), a 3-axial MEMS accelerometer (sampling frequency, $f_s = 32\,\text{Hz}$), an EDA sensor ($f_s = 4\,\text{Hz}$) and optical infrared thermometer ($f_s = 4\,\text{Hz}$).

This specific work was focused on the signal measured by the EDA sensor (see Table 1 for details). Regarding this sensor, the E4 device provides a way to measure the electrical conductance by passing a minuscule amount of current between two silver-coated electrodes in contact with the wrist skin, as they are located onto the device bracelet.

**Table 1.** Technical specification of the EDA sensor embedded in Empatica E4.

| Specification | Value |
|---|---|
| Sampling frequency ($f_s$) | 4 Hz |
| Resolution | 900 pS |
| Range | 0.01–100 μS |
| Alternating current (max 100 μA) frequency | 8 Hz |
| Time needed for automatic calibration | 15 s |

---

[1] https://www.empatica.com/en-eu/research/e4/.

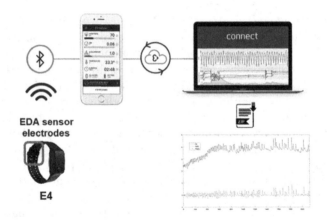

**Fig. 1.** Graphic representation of the IoT-enabled EDA measurements acquisition process. After the measuring session, data is retrieved through download from the Empatica cloud platform.

The E4 device can be used in two different modalities: streaming and recording mode, with the battery life declared as >20 h and >36 h, respectively. Herein, participants run the device in streaming mode allowing to monitor data in realtime from the mobile App (i.e., E4 realtime) over a Bluetooth Low Energy (BLE) connection. The EDA measurement and data acquisition process is graphically shown in Fig. 1. In order to access and download the recorded measurement data, the users shall create a personal account in the E4 Connect cloud-based repository, in which their own sessions are saved, including details about the duration, the device serial number, and the session date. Raw data can be downloaded as a compressed directory (.zip), containing one .csv file for each sensor and an additional file (named tags.csv) related to events marked during a session. Specifically, the EDA files are organised in single-column format, where the first row reports the starting time ($t_0$) of the data measurement process, the second shows the sampling rate, then measurement samples from the EDA sensor, giving skin conductance values in microSiemens ($\mu S$), are listed. Instead, in the tags.csv files each row represents the time instant in which the physical button located on the E4 has been pressed, expressed in UTC and synchronised with the acquisition start time $t_0$ specified in the other files, belonging to the same session.

### 3.2   Test Population and Data Collection

Seven healthy subjects, 2 males and 5 females of age (35.7 ± 17.9) years (mean ± standard deviation), were recruited. To gather their physiological measurement data, participants were submitted to six sessions of auditory stimulation: three sessions lasted 11 min and the remaining ones 12 min, as shown in Fig. 2. Specifically, in the first and last 5 min of each session, the subject's baseline (i.e., EDA data at resting condition) was acquired, while during the central minutes (i.e., 1 or 2 min) the physiological changes under acoustic stimuli were measured. In order to reduce possible distractions during sessions, the participants were left alone in their room, lying on a bed with closed eyes. The E4 was attached on the dominant wrist to acquire the skin electrical signal. Prior to signals registration, volunteers were asked to push the event-marker button of the wristband, at the start and at the end of the acoustic stimulus, thus allowing the real-time annotations of sessions.

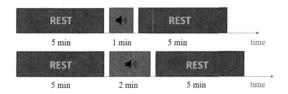

**Fig. 2.** Schematic representation of the temporal structure of the auditory stimulation sessions presented to the participants: 11 min (upper graph) and 12 min long (bottom graph).

To elicit emotions in volunteers, three audio clips were extracted from the IADS database, which includes a list of sounds categorised in terms of valence, arousal and dominance using the SAM scale. The three clips, lasting 6 s each, were selected considering the associated valence score: pleasant (no. 815: 'Rock-NRoll'), neutral (no. 722: 'Walking') and unpleasant (no. 275: 'Scream') sound. Table 2 lists the mean and standard deviation values of the three evaluation dimensions of each audio clip chosen from the IADS database, according to female and male subjects.

**Table 2.** Gender-based evaluation (mean ± standard deviation) of the stimuli (i.e. audio clips) chosen to elicit emotions in the volunteers, for each dimension.

| Gender | Sound | Valence | Arousal | Dominance |
|--------|-------|---------|---------|-----------|
| Female | RockNRoll | 8.13 ± 1.41 | 6.75 ± 2.28 | 6.99 ± 1.99 |
| | Walking | 5.02 ± 1.19 | 4.87 ± 1.86 | 4.85 ± 1.41 |
| | Scream | 1.65 ± 1.16 | 8.35 ± 1.32 | 2.11 ± 1.74 |
| Male | RockNRoll | 7.56 ± 1.65 | 7.00 ± 1.77 | 6.67 ± 2.00 |
| | Walking | 4.61 ± 1.22 | 5.08 ± 2.00 | 4.45 ± 1.56 |
| | Scream | 2.49 ± 1.94 | 7.96 ± 1.67 | 3.04 ± 2.19 |

Previous studies, such as Akdermir et al. [17], found that stimuli lasting from 2 to 4 min are useful to produce variations of physiological parameters, including the EDA. Therefore, in this study, two playlists with different length were created for each sound, to investigate the effect of the stimulus duration on the elicited physiological changes. Given the fact that audio clips in the IADS database are only 6 s long, in the first playlist the same clip was reproduced ten times, thus obtaining a 1 min-long stimulus, while in the second playlist the audio clip was repeated twenty times, in order to reach a total duration of 2 min. This way, the 2 min-long audio clip allowed to replicate the procedure used in [17]; the 1 min-long clip was added in order to check whether the repetition of the same sound may affect or not the subjects' reaction.

Based on the subjective assessment of sound, the presented audio tracks can elicit different emotions in different individuals. Hence, to measure the emotional response after each sound, participants were provided with the standardised SAM scale to identify themselves with the five different pictographs (scoring from 1 to 9) along the three dimensions. Such scores were compared with the standardised values provided by the IADS database, to investigate whether the experience from our participants was consistent or not with the standardised ranges.

## 4    Data Processing

In order to accurately analyse the SCR as a reaction to the stimulus, raw data were analysed in time domain, not by resorting to automatic tools (such as LedaLAB[2]) but following the standard procedure described by iMotions [12]. First of all, data from the first and last 4 s within the trials were discarded to remove the artefacts (e.g., transient noise due to the movement of the subjects during the recordings, mostly at the beginning and at the end of each session). Secondly, scanning each signal sample by sample, as in a sliding-window filter, the median EDA was computed for each sample and the surrounding samples in a window of 4 s, centred on the current sample. Such median filter allowed to decompose the phasic component from the EDA signal, and peak-related features were extracted [1,12]. In this sense, we use the phasic component as representing the signal physiological content, and the number of peaks as a meaningful feature to represent the effects of an external stimulus [18], and thus to compare the reaction to different stimuli of a same subject, or to the same stimulus by different people. According to literature [10], a peak-and-through detection algorithm has been developed to identify two thresholds of the SCR curve: the onsets at $TH_{on} = 0.01$ $\mu$S and offset at $TH_{off} = 0$ $\mu$S. Therefore, an onset was identified when SCR $> TH_{on}$ and an offset when SCR $< TH_{off}$. Then, back to the original EDA signal, for each onset-offset couple, the exact position of each peak was identified and counted as peak. An example is shown in Fig. 3.

---

[2] http://www.ledalab.de/.

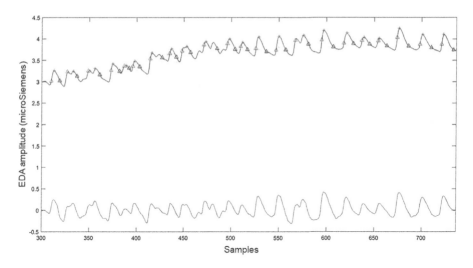

**Fig. 3.** Example of raw EDA signal (blue) with onsets (green), peaks (yellow) and offsets (red) marked. The SCR signal is in red. (Color figure online)

## 5  Results and Discussions

In the following sections, the findings from the proposed algorithm described in Sect. 4 are reported and discussed in detail, by comparing the results observed among the subjects involved and among the different acoustic stimuli.

### 5.1  Comparison Among Individuals

As explained in Sect. 3.2, each session was composed by three parts of different duration. For this reason, the number of EDA peaks per minute was defined (a kind of *peaks frequency*) as a representative metric and counted for each part, in order to understand how the peaks frequency changed during the music listening phase, and in the absence of acoustic stimuli phase, irrespective of the absolute time duration of each phase. Graphs in Fig. 4 show the results of the peaks frequency analysis, with values obtained by averaging the outcomes on the three sessions. For each subject, the orange bar represents the peaks frequency in the first 5 min of acquisition at rest (i.e., pre-stimulus); the yellow bar indicates the rate of EDA peaks in the phase of external stimulation (i.e., stimulus), while the green bar states the number of peaks per minute computed in the last minutes, following the end of the sound clip (i.e., post-stimulus).

By comparing the three columns and the two rows in Fig. 4, especially focusing on the middle phase of acquisition, it is evident that the reaction determined by listening to different sounds is subjective. For example, by examining how much the pleasant sound affects the physiological changes in EDA properties, it is possible to notice that while the subjects S3, S4 and S5 are more sensitive to

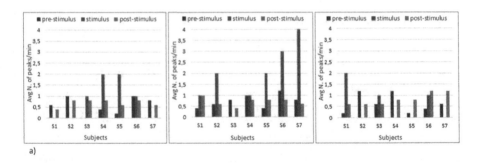

a)

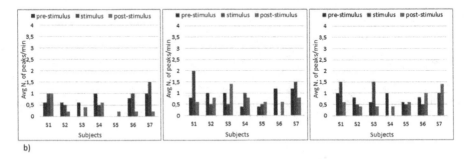

b)

**Fig. 4.** Average number of peaks per minute recorded on signal acquired during the listening of pleasant (first column), unpleasant (second column) and neutral (third column) sound for each subject: a) one-minute-long sound clip, b) two-minute-long sound clip.

sound clips lasting one minute, the subjects S1, S2, S6 and S7 are more sensitive to pleasant sound two minutes long. Regarding the effect of the unpleasant sound on the EDA signals, in one-minute-long sound clips, six out of seven participants, except S3, show a number of peaks per minute greater or equal to the one recorded during the resting phase (i.e., $\geq 1$). This illustrates an increase of the number of peaks per minute from the resting to the stimulating phase. However, when the stimulating period was longer (i.e., 2 min), the number of peaks per minute decreases drastically, even reaching zero for S4. Therefore the subjects S2, S5, S6 and S7 appear to be more sensitive to unpleasant sounds of short duration. Finally, the values obtained from the analysis of EDA signals measured during the listening to the neutral sound are interesting: four out of seven participants, namely S2, S4, S5 and S7, show an average peaks frequency that increases from 0 to higher values under longer stimuli. The opposite considerations can be applied to S6.

### 5.2    Comparison Among Different Acoustic Stimuli

In this section, the results obtained from the analysis of signals acquired during listening sessions of pleasant, neutral and unpleasant sounds are compared. In particular, the peaks rate was averaged over all the participants, in order to obtain a single value for each sound listened to, for both the sound clip lengths. Figure 5 displays the findings from acquisitions with the external stimuli lasting one minute (left side), and two minutes (right side).

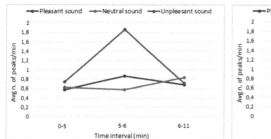
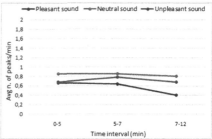

**Fig. 5.** Changes in average EDA peaks rate over all subjects: before, during and after the listening of pleasant (green line), neutral (blue line) and unpleasant (yellow line) sound clips, lasting one minute (left side) and two minutes (right side). (Color figure online)

According to the first analysis among the subjects, it is evident how the acoustic sounds produce different effects on the EDA signals of the listeners, depending on both the length and the valence score of the sound clip. Specifically, the unpleasant sound elicits a different effect depending on the time duration of the stimulus. Looking at the effects of unpleasant sound stimulus lasting one-minute, it is possible to see an increase of EDA peaks per minute during the period of sound listening, and then it returns close to starting values. However, slight changes and variations are observable in unpleasant sounds lasting two minutes, as well as when using neutral sounds as external stimulus.

In order to explore if the physiological response of the participants was somehow associated to the emotional experience, we compared the SAM scores declared by the participants, given in Table 3, and the number of peaks per minute counted from the EDA signals.

**Table 3.** Average scores of valence, arousal and dominance and related standard deviation for each sound clip listened, over all the tests participants.

| | Valence | Arousal | Dominance |
|---|---|---|---|
| RockNRoll | $7.1 \pm 0.8$ | $6.9 \pm 0.7$ | $6.5 \pm 1.1$ |
| Walking | $5.3 \pm 0.5$ | $4.0 \pm 0.9$ | $5.1 \pm 1.5$ |
| Scream | $2.3 \pm 0.8$ | $6.7 \pm 0.9$ | $3.1 \pm 1.1$ |

The values rated by subjects involved in our experimental test are comparable to the standardised scores in IADS database: the 'RockNRoll' and 'Scream' sounds were evaluated as arousing, while the 'Walking' as a relaxing sound. Even though both the pleasant and unpleasant sounds have a high and quite similar arousal score, 'Scream' was assessed with a low value of valence, that corresponds to an unhappy emotional state according to the SAM scale. Regarding the dominance and control dimensions, the 'Scream' elicited subjects feeling dominated and dependent on the sound, the 'RockNRoll' sound produces a sensation of maximum control in the situation, while the 'Walking' sound was rated as neutral.

# 6    Conclusion

EDA (or equivalenty GSR) is a biometric signal reflecting changes in the electrical properties of the skin, produced by external emotional stimuli [23]. In this work, the EDA signal was measured by using the E4 wristband and then processed in time domain, by evaluating the effects of different type and length of acoustic stimuli, in a small population. In particular, the number of peaks per minute of the EDA curve was counted, being the event-related feature, and then compared among the subjects and among the stimuli. Regarding the unpleasant sound, the same effect (i.e. an increase of EDA peaks per minute during the listening period) in almost all individuals was presented especially for short sound, probably due to the track played: an unexpected and well-known annoying sound (i.e., 'Scream'). Probably, the negative emotion was able to induce a high sweat reaction, and consequently evident physiological changes. However the same reaction, if the external stimulus is too long, can be affected by the habituation phenomenon, resulting in a lower number of peaks per minute in the EDA curve. Contrarily, the findings from the pleasant and neutral stimuli are more randomly distributed. Many subjects did not show any physiological reaction to 'Walking' and 'RockNRoll' sounds, especially when presented the one-minute-long tracks.

In general, the results confirm that the physiological changes in EDA are visible, but subjective. Even though different individuals can share some emotional status or mental perception of the same sound track (as declared in SAM scale scores), their physiological features can have significant differences. This statement is evident for pleasant sound, where high perception of affective valence and intensity corresponds to a small number of peaks during the stimulation. Contrarily, the low valence and high arousal of 'Scream' sound can be strictly associated to the bigger number of peaks during the elicitation of an unpleasant experience.

Although the results of this preliminary experiment are promising, some clear limitations rely in the use of a single audio clip per IADS category, the small population affected by gender imbalance, and the use of the time-domain peak detection approach alone. More accurate findings can be achieved by enrolling a wider and more heterogeneous population in terms of gender and age. For example, the different perception of an external stimulus (e.g. acoustic), and consequently the resulting EDA fluctuations can be compared among males and females of different ages. Additionally, also selecting more sound tracks of the same valence scores from the IADS database, can allow to obtain more generalised and reliable findings. These activities are foreseen as future developments of the research.

# References

1. Bakker, J., Pechenizkiy, M., Sidorova, N.: What's your current stress level? Detection of stress patterns from GSR sensor data. In: IEEE 11th International Conference on Data Mining Workshops, pp. 573–580. IEEE (2011)
2. Bradley, M.M., Lang, P.J.: Measuring emotion: the self-assessment Manikin and the semantic differential. J. Behav. Ther. Exp. Psychiat. **25**(1), 49–59 (1994)
3. Bradley, M.M., Lang, P.J.: The international affective picture system (IAPS) in the study of emotion and attention. In: Series in Affective Science. Handbook of Emotion Elicitation and Assessment, pp. 29–46 (2007)
4. Can, Y.S.: How to relax in stressful situations: a smart stress reduction system. Healthcare **8**(2), 100 (2020)
5. Domínguez-Jiménez, J., Campo-Landines, K., Martínez-Santos, J., Delahoz, E., Contreras-Ortiz, S.: A machine learning model for emotion recognition from physiological signals. Biomed. Signal Process. Control **55**, 101646 (2020)
6. Dumitriu, T., Cémpanu, C., Ungureanu, F., Manta, V.: Experimental analysis of emotion classification techniques. In: IEEE 14th International Conference on Intelligent Computer Communication and Processing, pp. 63–70. IEEE (2018). https://doi.org/10.1109/ICCP.2018.8516647
7. Ekman, P., Levenson, R.W., Friesen, W.V.: Autonomic nervous system activity distinguishes among emotions. Science **221**(4616), 1208–10 (1983)
8. Empatica Inc., MI, IT: E4 WristBand from Empatica User's Manual (2018)
9. Pozzi, G., Sarti, A., Borrelli, C.: Music emotion detection. A framework based on electrodermal activities. http://hdl.handle.net/10589/152931. Accessed 30 Jun 2020
10. Gautam, A., Simoes-Capela, N., Schiavone, G., Acharyya, A., de Raedt, W., Van Hoof, C.: A data driven empirical iterative algorithm for GSR signal pre-processing. In: 2018 26th European Signal Processing Conference (EUSIPCO), pp. 1162–1166. IEEE (2018)
11. Hu, X., Li, F., Ng, T.D.J.: On the relationships between music-induced emotion and physiological signals. In: 19th International Society for Music Information Retrieval Conference (2018)
12. iMotions: Galvanic skin response (GSR): the complete pocket guide. https://imotions.com/blog/galvanic-skin-response/. Accessed 30 Jun 2020
13. Kim, J., Andre, E.: Emotion recognition based on physiological changes in music listening. IEEE Trans. Pattern Anal. Mach. Intell. **30**(12), 2067–2083 (2009)
14. Myroniv, B., Wu, C.W., Ren, Y., Christian, A., Bajo, E., Tseng, Y.C.: Analyzing user emotions via physiology signals. Data Sci. Pattern Recogn. **2**, 11–25 (2017)
15. Poh, M., Loddenkemper, T., Swenson, N.C., Goyal, S., Madsen, J.R., Picard, R.W.: Continuous monitoring of electrodermal activity during epileptic seizures using a wearable sensor. In: 2010 Annual International Conference of the IEEE Engineering in Medicine and Biology, pp. 4415–4418 (2010)
16. Prasomphan, S.: Detecting human emotion via speech recognition by using speech spectrogram. In: 2015 IEEE International Conference on Data Science and Advanced Analytics on Proceedings, pp. 1–10. IEEE (2015)

17. Saime, A., Sadık, K., Vedat, B.: Investigation into the effects of classical Turkish music on galvanic skin response and skin temperature of schizophrenic patients. J. Network. Technol. **1**(4), 181–188 (2010)

18. Singh, R.R., Conjeti, S., Banerjee, R.: A comparative evaluation of neural network classifiers for stress level analysis of automotive drivers using physiological signals. Biomed. Sig. Process. Control **8**(6), 740–754 (2013)

19. Smets, E., et al.: Comparison of machine learning techniques for psychophysiological stress detection. In: Serino, S., Matic, A., Giakoumis, D., Lopez, G., Cipresso, P. (eds.) MindCare 2015. CCIS, vol. 604, pp. 13–22. Springer, Cham (2016). https://doi.org/10.1007/978-3-319-32270-4_2

20. Soto, J.A.C., Levenson, R.W.: Emotion recognition across cultures: the influence of ethnicity on empathic accuracy and physiological linkage. Emotion **9**(6), 874–884 (2010)

21. Topoglu, Y., Watson, J., Suri, R., Ayaz, H.: Electrodermal activity in ambulatory settings: a narrative review of literature. In: Ayaz, H. (ed.) AHFE 2019. AISC, vol. 953, pp. 91–102. Springer, Cham (2020). https://doi.org/10.1007/978-3-030-20473-0_10

22. Uhrig, M.K., et al.: Emotion elicitation: a comparison of pictures and films. Front. Psychol. **7**, 180 (2016)

23. Ultan Cowley, B., Torniainen, J.: A short review and primer on electrodermal activity in human computer interaction applications. arXiv preprint arXiv-1608 (2016)

24. Williams, D., Wu, C.Y., Hodge, V., Murphy, D., Cowling, P.: A psychometric evaluation of emotional responses to horror music. In: AES (ed.) Audio Engineering Society: 146th International Pro Audio Convention (2019)

25. Wu, Y., Liu, Y., Su, N., Ma, S., Ou, W.: Predicting online shopping search satisfaction and user behaviors with electrodermal activity. In: Proceedings of the 26th International Conference on World Wide Web Companion, WWW 2017 Companion, International World Wide Web Conferences Steering Committee, Republic and Canton of Geneva, CHE, pp. 855–856 (2017). https://doi.org/10.1145/3041021.3054226

26. Yang, W., et al.: Affective auditory stimulus database: an expanded version of the international affective digitized sounds (IADS-E). Behav. Res. Methods **50**, 1415–1429 (2018)

27. Zhao, B., Wang, Z., Yu, Z., Guo, B.: EmotionSense: emotion recognition based on wearable wristband. In: 2018 IEEE SmartWorld, Ubiquitous Intelligence Computing, Advanced Trusted Computing, Scalable Computing Communications, Cloud Big Data Computing, Internet of People and Smart City Innovation, pp. 346–355. IEEE (2018). https://doi.org/10.1109/SmartWorld.2018.00091

# Scenarios and Security

# CoviHealth: A Pilot Study with Teenagers in Schools of Centre of Portugal

María Vanessa Villasana[1(✉)], Ivan Miguel Pires[2,3,4], Juliana Sá[1,5], Nuno M. Garcia[2], Eftim Zdravevski[6], Ivan Chorbev[6], and Petre Lameski[6]

[1] Faculty of Health Sciences, Universidade da Beira Interior, 6200-506 Covilhã, Portugal
maria.vanessa.villasana.abreu@ubi.pt, julianasa@fcsaude.ubi.pt
[2] Instituto de Telecomunicações, Universidade da Beira Interior, 6200-001 Covilhã, Portugal
impires@it.ubi.pt, ngarcia@di.ubi.pt
[3] Computer Science Departement, Polytechnic Institute of Viseu, 3504-510 Viseu, Portugal
[4] UICISA:E Research Centre, School of Health, Polytechnic Institute of Viseu, 3504-510 Viseu, Portugal
[5] Hospital Center of Cova da Beira, 6200-251 Covilhã, Portugal
[6] Faculty of Computer Science and Engineering, University Ss Cyril and Methodius, 1000 Skopje, North Macedonia
{eftim.zdravevski,ivan.chorbev,petre.lameski}@finki.ukim.mk

**Abstract.** Obesity is one of the most common problem that can be avoid with the correct education of the teenagers. There are different methods, but the use of the mobile devices to promote the creation of social challenges is important, because the teenagers act mainly in groups. The use of questionnaires, challenges and gamification purposes may promote the use of this type of mobile applications by teenagers. It is a special population that needs the adoption of different interactive technologies. The studies available are not validated by healthcare professionals. First of all, we started to analyze the related work of obesity problem, mobile applications, and different methodologies adopted with teenagers. By the end, seven students participated in the study with the performance of visualization of daily tips and curiosities, answering questionnaires, monitoring of physical activity and gamification. The teenagers were satisfied with the strategies adopted, but this study was affected by the pandemic situation around the world. In general, the participants were satisfied with the use of the mobile, and they would like to use it in the future for the improvement of their nutrition and physical activity habits.

**Keywords:** Teenagers · Mobile application · Nutrition · Physical activity · Health · Education

## 1 Introduction

Nowadays, it was verified that the teenagers have an inadequate and little knowledge about healthy nutrition and physical activity. They spend a lot of time with technological

© ICST Institute for Computer Sciences, Social Informatics and Telecommunications Engineering 2021
Published by Springer Nature Switzerland AG 2021. All Rights Reserved
R. Goleva et al. (Eds.): HealthyIoT 2020, LNICST 360, pp. 139–147, 2021.
https://doi.org/10.1007/978-3-030-69963-5_10

equipment and did not practice physical activity [1, 2]. It causes different healthcare problems in the teenagers, including the obesity [3–5]. One of the factors for the poor habits of the teenagers are socioeconomic factors [6]. Still, the reduces physical activity and the energy intake is other important factor in this type of population [5].

The obesity is caused by the excessive body fat with the difference between energy expenditure and calories intake [7]. It caused the development of several diseases, including hyperglycemia, dyslipidemia, hypertriglyceridemia, low levels of High-Density Lipoprotein, and hypertension [8]. However, the performance of physical activity is the best method to spend calories and control the weight [9].

The prevalence and incidence of obesity and overweight in teenagers was proposed in the National Health Plan - Review and Extension to 2020 [10]. Portugal is not exception, and the National Program for the Promotion of Healthy Eating was created to promote the combat of the obesity. One of the strategies that Portugal adopted was to attempt to increase the levels of physical activity in young people and teenagers [11].

A Body Mass Index (BMI) for age with more than a typical deviation above the median established in child growth patterns and obesity as being higher than two standard deviations above the norm established in child growth patterns was created by the World Health Organization (WHO) for individuals aged between 5 and 19 years old [7]. This population is considered as overweight between the 85th and 95th percentile, and obese above the 95th percentile [12]. Thus, the WHO verified, in 2016, that the number of teenagers that are overweight or obese exceeded 340 millions of individuals [7].

The purpose of this study is to use a mobile application for the promotion of healthy nutrition and physical activity habits by teenagers during a trial of five weeks. During the time of the study, different tips, curiosities, challenges, and questionnaires were proposed for the seven teenagers that participated in the study. The teenagers were aged between 13 and 16 years old, and they are students in the public schools in the Covilhã, and Fundão municipalities (Portugal) [14]. The mobile application includes different methodologies to captivate the attention of the teenagers, and it also includes methods to stimulate the physical activity. The gamification, personalized messages, and medical control are some of the methodologies implemented. The teenagers answered different questionnaires about physical activity and nutrition during the study. The analysis of the different answers was performed to evaluate the knowledge level of the teenagers.

This study revealed that the use of a mobile application is a good method to promote health nutrition and physical activity habits in teenagers. It was also verified that these population valued gamification techniques and the medical control. The effects of the use of mobile application should be reevaluated after the pandemic situation.

This paragraph and the introductory section. Section 2 presents the related work about the obesity, mobile applications for nutrition and physical activity and different methodologies used with this population. The methodology of CoviHealth project is presented in Sect. 3. Next, Sect. 4 presented the analysis of the initial questionnaire, the answers in the questionnaires about nutrition and physical activity, and the feedback questionnaire. The discussion of this study, and comparison with other studies are presented in Sect. 5. The conclusions are presented in Sect. 6.

## 2  Related Work

Obesity is considered a chronic, complex and multifactorial disease that is unfavorable for health, being characterized by an excessive increase in body fat that results from the imbalance of caloric expenditure and energy intake [7]. This imbalance is favorable to the development of several metabolic complications, namely insulin resistance, which leads to hyperglycemia, dyslipidemia, namely hypertriglyceridemia and low levels of High Density Lipoprotein (HDL), and arterial hypertension [8], also affecting the intestinal microbiota [15] that results from the interaction of several genetic, environmental and lifestyle factors [16].

The reduction and control of the incidence and prevalence of overweight and obesity in the child and school population is one of the goals proposed for 2020 in the National Health Plan - Review and Extension to 2020 [10]. Thus, in Portugal, the Directorate-General for Health created the National Program for the Promotion of Healthy Eating, in which public health strategies for combating obesity are addressed and created.

For children, adolescents and young adults between 5 and 19 years old, the World Health Organization (WHO) defines excess weight as the Body Mass Index (BMI) for age with more than a typical deviation above the median established in HDL child growth patterns. In turn, obesity is defined as being greater than 2 typical deviations above the median established in child growth patterns [7]. Thus, children, adolescents and young adults aged 13 to 19 between the 85th and 95th percentiles are overweight. It is further mentioned that with a percentile higher than the 95th percentile, they are classified as obese [12].

In 2018, the study [17], which presents data collected between 2015 and 2016 in Portugal, concludes that the prevalence of obesity increases with increasing age, being less prevalent in children and higher in the elderly. There are 3 inflection points in the prevalence of obesity throughout life, being them at 5, at 15 and, finally, at 75 years old. This study resulted in approximately 17.3% of children, under the age of 10 years, having pre-obesity and 23.6% of adolescents, aged between 10 and 18 years, having pre-obesity. 7.7% of children and 8.7% of adolescents were obese.

In 2017, the WHO estimates that, as adolescents are older, the level of physical activity decreases [18]. However, when analyzing the answers related to the question related to the accomplishment of "at least one hour of moderate to vigorous activity every day", this was performed by 25% of the children of 11 years, but for those of 15 years, the number drops to 16% [18]. The authors also conclude that the probability of sedentary behavior increases with age, with only 50% of 11-year-old children reporting watching 2 or more hours of television during the week, against 63% of those who are older [18].

In order to understand what type of functionalities are the most frequently present in mobile applications aimed at nutrition, physical activity and health, in the general population, a search was carried out in the Google Play Store, since the mobile application would be developed for the Android operating system [19]. The following keywords "nutrition", "diet", "calories", "health", "exercise" and "weight" were used for this search. 250 applications resulted from this search [19]. Thus, only 73 were analyzed, where the remaining were excluded by previously defined criteria [19]. The 73 applications were classified, verifying that most of them corresponds to applications related to "diet and nutrition" (52%) [19]. The remaining mobile applications are distributed by "health"

(25%), "physical activity" (12%) and education (11%) [19]. We also analyzed and categorized the different functionalities, including "diet", "anthropometric parameters", "social", "physical activity", "medical parameters", and, "vital parameters" [19]. From the study of the 73 mobile applications, we verified that the most features encountered in the mobile applications were weight, height, age, gender, objectives, calculation of calories needed, diet diary, database of food and calories, calories burned and calculation of intake of calories [19].

Finally, in order to discover the most used methodologies to obtain the participation and attention of young people with the use of mobile applications to improve health, a search for different studies was made. A search was made in different digital libraries, such as Springer, IEEE Xplore, and PubMed. Initially, we found 13,218 articles, where, after the exclusions, 9 articles were remaining due to the criteria that we established previously. These studies indicate the different techniques to attract the attention of young people, where, generally, it includes questionnaires and gamification techniques. The different features used in the different studies include the paper diary, the digital diet diary, the digital exercise diary, the use of notifications, the diet plan, the record of physical activity, the use of photos, the use of games, and the use of SMS.

## 3 Methods

Before this study, a methodology was proposed with the use of a mobile application [14], which was built with the aim of monitoring, advising and educating young people about health. This mobile application was named as CoviHealth, where young people could register their diet, physical activity, medication plans, anthropometric data, alerts and objectives. In addition, the teenagers could accept the challenges related to physical activity and fill the weekly questionnaires. The main screen will show a daily curiosity/suggestion related to nutrition and physical activity, and their effects on health.

As the project was developed in Covilhã, Portugal, two schools were proposed to collaborate, such as Escola Quinta das Palmeiras (Covilhã), and Escola Secundária com 3° Ciclo Ensino Básico do Fundão (Fundão). The selected students were aged between 13 and 18 years old, where 68 were selected from Fundão, and 105 were selected from Covilhã.

Between the 173 students, only 155 of them were validated, because the remaining reported an invalid email or they do not have a smartphone with Android operating system. During the study 28 students downloaded the mobile application from Google Play Store, where one was excluded by age range and execution of the questionnaires in the mobile application.

All validated students used the mobile application for 5 weeks, where 18 curiosities and 10 suggestions related to nutrition or physical activity were presented. In addition, 6 challenges in relation to the number of steps and calories were provided. Thus, 4 questionnaires related to the curiosities and suggestions provided were presented to the teenager.

At the end of the first five weeks, the mobile application was evaluated by the teenager with a questionnaire. All questionnaires were statistically analyzed by quantitative and qualitative variables. Finally, the analysis was performed by groups, applying the Chi-square test with the contingency tables.

# 4   Results

## 4.1   Sample Analysis

The population included in the study tries to have equivalent number of people from different genders, where the population has 14 of female gender, and 12 of male gender. In addition, the individuals are distributed by different ages, *i.e.,* between 13 and 18 years old.

In this study is also studied the presence of pathologies in the different subjects, where only 19% of teenagers reported that have some diseases, but only 8% reported that are taking some medication.

The different teenagers have between 1.43 m and 1.87 m of height, but they have major incidence between 1.60 m and 1.70 m of height. Related to the weight, they reported that have between 35 kg and 80 kg, but they have major incidence between 40 kg and 50 kg. Thus, it is possible to calculate the Body Mass Index (BMI) with these values, reporting that 67% reported the normal level of BMI, *i.e.,* between 18.5 and 24.9.

## 4.2   Analysis of Population Habits

In relation to the sleeping habits, most of the students are sleeping between 8 and 9 hours per night, and the majority is not consuming alcoholic beverages. Fortunately, 65% of analyzed teenagers practice sports, but only 62% are frequenting the gymnasium, where also 62% of teenagers practice exercise during 1 or 2 h for each day. Regarding the sports played, 39% of the teenagers play football, and 23% of the teenagers play basketball. Regarding the group sports, 35% of students prefer individual sports, and 31% of teenagers prefer team sports.

In general, the teenagers involved in the study did not have specific diet, where only 62% of individuals are consuming one or two pieces of fruit per day. However, only 4% are consuming candies between 5 to 6 times a week. In contrast, 54% of teenagers are drinking only between 0.5 L and 1 L of water per day.

## 4.3   Analysis of Weekly Questionnaires

The participants had available in the mobile application 4 weekly questionnaires, answered by the end of each week of the study and they are related to the different tips and curiosities presented during each week. Table 1 shows the answers on the different questionnaires. The correct answers are highlighted in Table 1.

Regarding the different questionnaires, in average, 54% of the answers of the questionnaire 1 are correct, 39.75% of the answers in the questionnaire 2 are correct, 73% of the answers in the questionnaire 3 are correct, and 50% of the answers in the questionnaire 4 are correct.

**Table 1.** Different answers of the different questionnaires.

| Questionnaires | Questions | Answer 1 | Answer 2 | Answer 3 | Answer 4 |
|---|---|---|---|---|---|
| 1 | 1 | 13% | 20% | 47% | 20% |
|   | 2 | 13% | 7% | 7% | 73% |
|   | 3 | 60% | 40% | - | - |
|   | 4 | 60% | 13% | 7% | 20% |
| 2 | 1 | 42% | 17% | 8% | 33% |
|   | 2 | 25% | 42% | 17% | 17% |
|   | 3 | 58% | 42% | - | - |
|   | 4 | 25% | 8% | 42% | 25% |
| 3 | 1 | 8% | 92% | 0% | 0% |
|   | 2 | 0% | 17% | 17% | 67% |
|   | 3 | 17% | 8% | 75% | 0% |
|   | 4 | 0% | 58% | 25% | 17% |
| 4 | 1 | 14% | 43% | 0% | 43% |
|   | 2 | 43% | 0% | 57% | 0% |
|   | 3 | 29% | 29% | 29% | 14% |
|   | 4 | 14% | 14% | 0% | 71% |

### 4.4 Analysis of Feedback Questionnaire

Related to the monitoring of physical activity components of the mobile application, the users are mainly satisfied with the different functionalities, but most of the students that answered the questionnaire said that they maintained the level of physical activity during the study. In addition, most of the teenagers are satisfied with the use of the training plan functionality. Related to the food, most of the students maintained their food habits.

Related to the educational features, the use of tips and curiosities are useful for most of the students, and the use of questionnaires are mainly reasonably useful to the improvement of the knowledge about education of nutrition and physical activity. In general, most of the students answered that the use of gamification motivated the use of the mobile application. The mobile application also allows the medical control, where most of the teenagers said that it is important.

In general, people are reasonably satisfied with the mobile application, and a large part of the students involved in the study said that will use the proposed mobile application.

## 5   Discussion

Due to the presence of similar studies in the literature, the results obtained by our study can be discussed with them. The CoviHealth project was implemented for 5 weeks, and only one study found was implemented in the same number of weeks and a similar number of teenagers [20]. *Spook et al.* [21] and Reid *et al.* [22] are two studies implemented during only one week. In [23], a larger number of teenagers participated in the study during only 4 weeks. Finally, Lee *et al.* [24] performed a study with a similar number of teenagers than CoviHealth project for 12 weeks.

It was verified that one study improved the diet of the teenagers with mobile applications [20]. Still, the dietary habits did not changed in the study [23]. The satisfaction with the methodology implemented was higher in the study [25]. However, in the study [24], the teenagers are clearly satisfied, and, in study [23], the teenagers are not satisfied. Regarding our study, the majority of the teenagers agreed to the use of mobile applications. Thus, similarly to our study, in [21], the teenagers said that they would continue using the mobile application.

Therefore, the use of mobile applications by teenagers is not recommended until between 14 and 16 years old [26], and we need to act in earlier age to promote healthier habits. The technological equipment, chu as mobile devices, is a good manner to prometon good habits in the different communities of teenagers.

The technology allows the healthcare professionals to monitor the teenagers anywhere, and it can be explained to the teenager in a consultation. Different validated methods are important to captivate the attention of the teenagers, including the pedometer, and the measurement of the energy expenditure [27–30].

Finally, CoviHealth project demonstrated that the use of a mobile application increases the good habits for physical activity and nutrition. However, this study was implemented in a pandemic situation and it affected the results obtained as well as the low number of teenagers that completed the study. The main limitation was that the mobile application was only focused in nutrition and physical activity. The technologies captivate this type of population.

## 6   Conclusions

The CoviHealth application intends to educate the teenagers about physical activity and nutrition with daily tips and curiosities, questionnaires, gamification, challenges, and other functionalities. The teenagers win points with the use of the mobile application to earn discounts in different stores.

At the beginning this study involved 26 teenagers, but we only analyzed the seven teenagers that finalized the study. The analyzed teenagers are aged between 13 and 16 years old, and they answered the feedback questionnaire. The study has the duration of five weeks with the availability of four weekly questionnaires about the tips and curiosities provided by the mobile application.

Regarding the different functionalities of the mobile application, the teenagers are mainly satisfied with the physical activity monitoring, tips and curiosities, and questionnaires. By the way, they choose the medical control as a relevant feature, and they indicated that the gamification functionalities motivated the use of the mobile application.

It was concluded that the use of the mobile application for the promotion of healthy nutrition and physical activity habits is reliable. However, due to the pandemic situation, this study should be performed with a more diverse population and an larger samples in the analysis.

**Acknowledgements.** This work is funded by FCT/MEC through national funds and co-funded by FEDER – PT2020 partnership agreement under the project **UIDB/EEA/50008/2020** (*Este trabalho é financiado pela FCT/MEC através de fundos nacionais e cofinanciado pelo FEDER, no âmbito do Acordo de Parceria PT2020 no âmbito do projeto UIDB/EEA/50008/2020*).

This work is also funded by National Funds through the FCT - Foundation for Science and Technology, I.P., within the scope of the project UIDB/00742/2020.

The work presented in this paper is also supported by the University of Sts. Cyril and Methodius in Skopje, Faculty of Computer Science and Engineering.

This article is based upon work from COST Action IC1303–AAPELE–Architectures, Algorithms and Protocols for Enhanced Living Environments and COST Action CA16226–SHELD-ON–Indoor living space improvement: Smart Habitat for the Elderly, supported by COST (European Cooperation in Science and Technology). More information in www.cost.eu.

Furthermore, we would like to thank the Politécnico de Viseu for their support.

# References

1. Harris, J., Cale, L., Duncombe, R., Musson, H.: Young people's knowledge and understanding of health, fitness and physical activity: issues, divides and dilemmas. Sport. Educ. Soc. **23**, 407–420 (2018). https://doi.org/10.1080/13573322.2016.1228047
2. Chen, A., Hancock, G.R.: Conceptualizing a theoretical model for school-centered adolescent physical activity intervention research. Quest **58**, 355–376 (2006). https://doi.org/10.1080/00336297.2006.10491887
3. Triches, R.M., Giugliani, E.R.J.: Obesity, eating habits and nutritional knowledge among school children. Revista de Saúde Pública **39**, 541–547 (2005). https://doi.org/10.1590/S0034-89102005000400004
4. Bhargava, M., Pracheth, R.: Physical activity and sedentary lifestyle towards teenagers' overweight/obesity status. Int. J. Community Med. Public Heal. **3**, 988 (2016). https://doi.org/10.18203/2394-6040.ijcmph20160942
5. Reilly, J.J., Kelly, J.: Long-term impact of overweight and obesity in childhood and adolescence on morbidity and premature mortality in adulthood: systematic review (2011). https://pubmed.ncbi.nlm.nih.gov/20975725/
6. Lenthe, F.J., et al.: Preventing socioeconomic inequalities in health behaviour in adolescents in Europe: background, design and methods of project TEENAGE. BMC Public Health **9**(1), 1–10 (2009). https://doi.org/10.1186/1471-2458-9-125
7. WHO: Obesity and overweight. https://www.who.int/en/news-room/fact-sheets/detail/obesity-and-overweight
8. Alberti, K.G.M.M., Zimmet, P., Shaw, J.: The metabolic syndrome—a new worldwide definition. Lancet **366**, 1059–1062 (2005). https://doi.org/10.1016/S0140-6736(05)67402-8
9. WHO: Adolescent obesity and related behaviours : trends and inequalities in the WHO European region 2002–2014. Copenhagen (2017)
10. Ministério da Saúde: Plano nacional de saúde: Revisão e extensão a 2020. Direção-Geral da Saúde 38 (2015)
11. Direcção-Geral da Saúde [DGS]: Programa Nacional Para a Promoção da Atividade Física - Portugal 2019. https://www.dgs.pt/portal-da-estatistica-da-saude/diretorio-de-informacao/diretorio-de-informacao/por-anos-dos-dados-1122895-pdf.aspx?v=%3D%3DDwAAAB%2BLCAAAAAAABAArySzItzVUy81MsTU1MDAFAHzFEfkPAAAA
12. Silva, F., Ferreira, E., Gonçalves, R., Cavaco, A.: Pediatric obesity: the reality of one consultation. Acta Med. Port. **25**, 91–96 (2012)
13. Wijnhoven, T.M.A., et al.: WHO European childhood obesity surveillance initiative 2008: weight, height and body mass index in 6–9-year-old children. Pediatr. Obes. **8**, 79–97 (2013). https://doi.org/10.1111/j.2047-6310.2012.00090.x

14. Villasana, M.V., et al.: CoviHealth: novel approach of a mobile application for nutrition and physical activity management for teenagers. In: ACM International Conference Proceeding Series, pp. 261–266. ACM, New York (2019)
15. Eckburg, P.B., et al.: Diversity of the human intestinal microbial flora. Science (80-) **308**, 1635–1638 (2005). https://doi.org/10.1126/science.1110591
16. Pérez-Herrera, A., Cruz-López, M.: Childhood obesity: current situation in Mexico. Nutr. Hosp. **36**, 463–469 (2019). https://doi.org/10.20960/nh.2116
17. Oliveira, A., et al.: Prevalence of general and abdominal obesity in Portugal: comprehensive results from the national food, nutrition and physical activity survey 2015–2016. BMC Public Health **18**, 614 (2018). https://doi.org/10.1186/s12889-018-5480-z
18. Nielsen, H., Bronwen Players, K.M.: Adolescent Health and Development in the WHO European Region: Can we do better?. https://www.euro.who.int/__data/assets/pdf_file/0005/407 219/AA-HA-adaptation-V7_maket_10.07.19_e_book_2.pdf?ua=1
19. Villasana, M.V., et al.: Mobile applications for the promotion and support of healthy nutrition and physical activity habits: a systematic review, extraction of features and taxonomy proposal. Open Bioinf. J. **13**, 50–71 (2019). https://doi.org/10.2174/1874196701907010050
20. Jimoh, F., et al.: Comparing diet and exercise monitoring using smartphone app and paper diary: a two-phase intervention study. JMIR mHealth uHealth. **6**, e17 (2018). https://doi.org/10.2196/mhealth.7702
21. Spook, J.E., Paulussen, T., Kok, G., Van Empelen, P.: Monitoring dietary intake and physical activity electronically: feasibility, usability, and ecological validity of a mobile-based ecological momentary assessment tool. J. Med. Internet Res. **15**, e214 (2013). https://doi.org/10.2196/jmir.2617
22. Reid, S.C., Kauer, S.D., Dudgeon, P., Sanci, L.A., Shrier, L.A., Patton, G.C.: A mobile phone program to track young people's experiences of mood, stress and coping. Soc. Psychiat. Psychiatr. Epidemiol. **44**, 501–507 (2009). https://doi.org/10.1007/s00127-008-0455-5
23. De Cock, N., et al.: Feasibility and impact study of a reward-based mobile application to improve adolescents' snacking habits. Public Health Nutr. **21**, 2329–2344 (2018). https://doi.org/10.1017/S1368980018000678
24. Lee, J.-E., Song, S., Ahn, J., Kim, Y., Lee, J.: Use of a mobile application for self-monitoring dietary intake: feasibility test and an intervention study. Nutrients **9**, 748 (2017). https://doi.org/10.3390/nu9070748
25. Lubans, D.R., Smith, J.J., Skinner, G., Morgan, P.J.: Development and implementation of a smartphone application to promote physical activity and reduce screen-time in adolescent boys. Front. Public Health **2**, 42 (2014). https://doi.org/10.3389/fpubh.2014.00042
26. Ertemel, A.V., Ari, E.: A marketing approach to a psychological problem: problematic smartphone use on adolescents. Int. J. Environ. Res. Public Health **17**, 2471 (2020). https://doi.org/10.3390/ijerph17072471
27. Pires, I.M., Felizardo, V., Pombo, N., Drobics, M., Garcia, N.M., Flórez-Revuelta, F.: Validation of a method for the estimation of energy expenditure during physical activity using a mobile device accelerometer. J. Ambient Intell. Smart Environ. **10**, 315–326 (2018). https://doi.org/10.3233/AIS-180494
28. Pires, I.M.S.: Aplicação móvel e plataforma Web para suporte à estimação do gasto energético em atividade física (2012). https://ubibliorum.ubi.pt/bitstream/10400.6/3721/1/dissertacao_Ivan.Pires.pdf
29. Quiala Cutiño, W.: Diseño de podómetro en dispositivo móvil: el i-Walker (2013)
30. Ugave, V.A., Anderson, C., Roy, S.: Smart indoor localization using machine learning techniques. Colorado State University. Libraries (2014)

# Dynamic Time Division Scheduling Protocol for Medical Application Using Frog Synchronization Algorithm

Norhafizah Muhammad and Tiong Hoo Lim$^{(\boxtimes)}$

Universiti Teknologi Brunei, Gadong, Brunei
norhafizah.muhammad@utb.edu.bn, lim.tiong.hoo@utb.edu.bn

**Abstract.** Different wireless sensing methods have been proposed for acquisition and measurement of body signals. In medical healthcare, it is critical that data are received simultaneously, processed, and analyzed in order to diagnose the disease accurately. For instance, to detect a patient with sleep apnea, it is necessary for the biosignals from dozens of biosensors including electroencephalography (EEG), electrocardiogram (ECG), photoplethysmogram (PPG), and peripheral oxygen saturation (Sp$O_2$) to be received in sequence it is used for diagnosis. However, it is difficult to accurately received these signals as their measurement frequencies are different from each other. Precise synchronization of the heartbeat with other measuring cycles of each biosensor is a critical attribute for identifying the correlation of each biosignal. Carrier Sense Multiple Access with Collision Avoidance (CSMA/CA) used in existing body area networks to guarantee the precise synchronization of multi-biosignals. This paper addressed this issue by proposing a bio-inspired Dynamic Time Division Scheduling Protocol (D-TDSP) based on the Frog Calling Algorithm (FCA) to adjust the timing of data transmission and to guarantee the synchronization of the sensing and receiving of multi-biosignals. The accuracy of the proposed algorithm is compared with the CSMA/CA method using a TelosB and XM1000 sensor nodes.

**Keywords:** Frog Calling Algorithm · Bio-inspired · Biosensor · Synchronization · Transmission data · Health monitoring

## 1 Introduction

Medical devices in the wireless body sensor networks (WBSNs) can be broadly divided into wired and wireless. Wired medical devices have high precision, but they are inconvenient to wear, complicated, and difficult to use by individual patients. In contrast, wireless medical devices are usually worn by the patient in the form of wearable devices making it more popular to be used at home for medical physiological monitoring and diagnosis [1,8]. These devices can be

© ICST Institute for Computer Sciences, Social Informatics and Telecommunications Engineering 2021
Published by Springer Nature Switzerland AG 2021. All Rights Reserved
R. Goleva et al. (Eds.): HealthyIoT 2020, LNICST 360, pp. 148–161, 2021.
https://doi.org/10.1007/978-3-030-69963-5_11

added to the networks as new or additional biometric needs to be collected. WBSNs consist of a number of short-range wireless communication devices. The biosensor on each device periodically receives biometric signal data through the connected biosensors. The biosensor can be embedded within the communication devices, or implant or attached outside the human body [3]. Each device is placed near the human body to collect data such as electrocardiograms, heart rate, and acceleration.

Individual device periodically receives the biometric data from the biosensor and transmit the signal collected to a centralised server for processing. Each device can perform time synchronization using periodic biosignal generated from the individual nodes. To analyze different biosignals received from different biosensor for medical diagnosis, it is necessary to read those biosignals from one or several devices accuracy and periodically in a synchronised manner [2]. As the biosensor devices are attached at different body parts, signals arriving from several devices may not be synchronized with the measured time. According to Pflugradt et al. [7], biosignal measurements can be partially obstructed by environmental influences and motion artifacts as the patients are usually not at rest. Data acquisition devices like ECG and PPG sensors are can be disrupted due to contacts failure or shifting photosensor positions [7]. The presence of intermittent radio interference from other medical devices can also disrupt the bio-signal transmission of the nodes [6]. Hence, there is a need to develop a fault tolerance data transmission scheduling algorithm that can guarantee sensing data synchronization and sequencing to make accuracy medical diagnosis.

In this paper, a time division based scheduling algorithm is proposed that can adapt and adjust its firing time according to the environment without affecting the sensing data sequence and the synchronized transmission. The main contribution of this paper is the development and analysis of a novel Bio-inspired algorithm called Dynamic Time Division Scheduling Protocol (D-TDSP) for Wireless Biosensor Networks (WBN) that capture and transmit the biomedical signals according to actual diagnosis pathway for a disease. The D-TDSP dynamically allocated the transmission time for each node using a modified Time Division Multiple Access (TDMA) approaches based on Frog Calling Algorithms (FCA).

The analysis from hardware experimental results have shown that the proposed D-TDSP is tolerate to single point of failure as there is no centralised control on the transmission scheduling. Individual node can adjust its transmission period according to the transmission time of its neighboring nodes. The proposed algorithm can also adapt to network changes due to device addition, and node removal or temporary anomaly due to interference compare to Firefly Synchronization (FAST) or default CSMA/CA.

Section 2 presents the basic background on the works related to time synchronization and scheduling in WBSNs followed by the design of the proposed algorithm in Sect. 3. In Sect. 4, the scenario and experimental setup used for the evaluation of the proposed D-TDSP are described. Section 5 and 6 discusses and validates the results obtained from the hardware experiments using a combination of two types of nodes. In Sect. 7, we conclude with future research.

# 2   Remote Healthcare Diagnosis and Detection

The WBSN can be used to sense, monitor, capture and extract physiological information of a patient using biosensor such as the electroencephalography (EEG), electrocardiogram (ECG), photoplethysmogram (PPG), and peripheral oxygen saturation (SpO$_2$) [5]. They can also be used to assist in other aspects of a patient's care, such as reporting on the current real-time location of a patient, recording a patient's condition for later analysis, or communicating a patient's condition to a remote party, such as a hospital or physician. These biosensor node can be attached or implanted to the patient's body [10].

WBSN applications need to be easy to use and with minimal user configuration. The attached biosensors should not intervene with the patient daily activities. It should be able to deliver and manage the information related to the patient care remotely [8]. Each biosensor will have its own timing circuit with a local clock. The biosensor needs to be connected to the network and the communication timing between biosensor nodes need to be synchronized to transmit the biodata without interfering with another nodes.

Most of these functions require tight time synchronization to function properly especially for applications that require two or more parameters for diagnostic or treatment [9]. They usually involves time synchronization of multiple biosensors forming a dynamically network. These networks need to be reconfigurable automatically to allow the nodes to join or leave the network, or to overcome communication failure triggered by interference from other radio devices. Upon joining the network, each node in the WBSNs must synchronize with one another. This synchronization may account for a number of possible sources of time discrepancy, such as differences in time stamping, communications latency during signal transmittance and/or other sources.

## 2.1   Packet Synchronization in Medical Application

Time synchronization is critical for time-sensitive applications such as medical health [12] for diagnostic in an Artificial Intelligence based medical application [7]. Zong et al. [11] mentioned the applications of time synchronization can be collaborated, coordinated and localized the position of the nodes. They found out that these nodes require precise timing in order to cooperate and monitor the physical or environmental variables.

Fixed time synchronization algorithm has been used in the MAC layer to ensure that data can be collected and transmitted reliable at a predetermined interval. In fixed time synchronization, the transmission interval allocated to individual node is equally divided among a set of nodes within a time period. Each node will need to transmit at the assigned interval to avoid packet collisions using time division approaches. However, fixed time synchronization approach is not suitable for medical application as the sensing data needs to be transmitted at any time when a critical event is detected. The default CSMA/CA transmission protocol at the MAC layer is prone to collision when the number of biosensor nodes increases. Hence, there is a need to apply bio-inspired synchronization algorithm at the application layer to ensure that the patient physiological data can be received promptly and reliably.

## 2.2  Frog Calling Synchronization Algorithm

The bio-inspired, Frog Calling Algorithm (FCA) is a self-organized control algorithm. This synchronization is based on the calling behavior of the Japanese Frog developed and modeled by Aihara et al. [4]. The main purpose of this frog behavior is to attract the female frog. The process is when there is a group of male frogs in the area, when one start calling, the others will start calling too. With the multiple calling, the female frog will have difficulties to distinguish which male frog is calling. Hence, they shifted the time of their calling [4]. Aihara et al. [4] developed a self-organizing scheduling scheme inspired by FCA for collision-free transmission scheduling in Wireless Sensor Networks. The authors evaluated their proposed algorithm in simulation and the results have shown that it can reduce the data transmission failures and improves the data collection ratio up to 24% compared to a random transmission method.

# 3  Dynamic Time Division Scheduling Protocol

In this section presents the algorithm framework of the D-TDSP. The D-TDSP allows the nodes fired evenly distributed within a time period. In a network, there are a set of number of nodes which work in a single hop topology. Each of the node will have the same period of time, where in this case T = 32 kHz. Figure 1 below shows the process of the dynamic time division scheduling protocol approach.

Figure 1(a) shows the initial stage before the algorithm starts. All of the nodes seen are not in periodic and synchronized position. When node A fired, it will look for the previous node, which is node B and it will use the Eq. 1 to evaluate the new position. As soon as Node B jump to new position, B as shown in Fig. 1 (b) and consequently. This will be repeated with the other nodes. Each node will adjust its transmission position until all of the nodes are evenly spread within the length period of time of the basestation (as shown in Fig. 1(c) below).

$$f(x) = f^{-1}(f(t^{'}) - \epsilon) \tag{1}$$

The value of $\epsilon$ is determined by Eq. 2, the mathematical equation shown below.

$$\epsilon = (\frac{t^{''} + t^{'}}{2})\alpha \tag{2}$$

where *alpha* is a synchronization damping function.

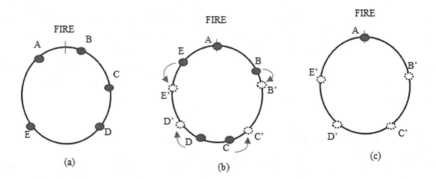

**Fig. 1.** Adaptive transmission scheduling algorithm (a) Node fires at a time period T. (b) Node responds to neighbors firing to adjust its firing timing between A and C

## 4    Experimental Setup

To evaluate the performance of D-TDSP against CSMA/CA random transmission and a firefly-inspired scheduling algorithm called Firefly Adaptive Scheduling Transmission (FAST), an xm1000 motes will be used as the WBN node. These nodes will be deployed in a similar manners to the application in the healthcare monitoring systems shown in Fig. 2. The bio sensors are to be attached on or implanted into the human body to collect physiological information such the electrocardiogram (ECG), electroencephalography (EEG), pulse rate, blood pressure, body temperature and $(SpO_2)$ and each biosensor will be connected to the XM1000 nodes. The WBSN will be operating in a star topology configuration, where all the data from the biosensor will be sent to the base station using single hop communications.

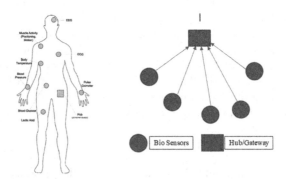

**Fig. 2.** The WBNs with biosensor attached to the body and a node to transmit the sensed data to the gateway.

A TelosB node will be used as a monitoring base station to collect the synchronization statistics and monitor the scheduling of the data transmission. XM1000 mote will be used as the individual sensor nodes that will collect the biodata to be transmitted within a clock cycle as shown in Fig. 3. Each nodes will have a unique id and the base station will need to capture the sequence and order of the packet received, and calculate the Packet Delivery Rate (PDR) using Eq. 3 below.

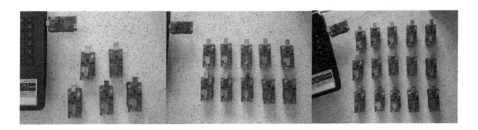

**Fig. 3.** The 5, 10, and 15 XM1000 nodes used for the experiment with one telosB mote connected to the notebook for data collection.

$$Packet\ Delivery\ Ratio, PDR = \frac{P_{rx} \times 100}{\sum_{i=1}^{n} P_{G(i)}} \tag{3}$$

Where $P_{rx}$ is the total number of data packets received by the sink node and $P_G$ is the packet generated by the source node.

Different numbers of 5, 10, 15 XM1000 motes were used to evaluate the scalability of the proposed algorithms as shown in Fig. 3. A laptop will be connected to the monitoring node to store and display the statistics collected. The synchronization process will begin when the first node starts to fire. The rest of the sensor nodes receiving the message will adjust its transmission period and transmit its own messages. This process will continue until the experiment ends.

Three set of experiments are conducted and repeated to compare the order of packet arrival at the base station and reliability in term of the PDR.

## 5    Results

In this section, the performance analysis of D-TDSP is compare against the random CSMA/CA and FAST. Three set of experiments are performed. The first experiment evaluates the sequencing of the packet received and the PDR against the network size for the three algorithms. The second and third experiments analyze the reliability of all the three algorithms when 1. a new node is added to the network and 2. When a node temporary fail to model scenario such as radio interference or node maintenance to replace battery.

## 5.1    Sequencing of Packet Delivered for 5 Nodes

In Fig. 4, Fig. 5 and Fig. 6 below show the synchronization process of the three synchronizations, the D-TDSP, FAST and CSMA/CA. It can be seen that the D-TDSP and FAST synchronization can achieved synchronization within the period of time as shown in Fig. 4 and Fig. 5 respectively. By observing the FAST synchronization process in Period 3, when all of the nodes transmitted it shows that the nodes were then in sleep mode for a short time before going into Period 4. In the D-TDSP, the nodes in Period 4 can be seen that it broadcasted the data in an evenly manners. While in CSMA/CA shown in Fig. 5 shows that the nodes transmit at a synchronicity patterns but the firing time will be at random and the nodes will only fire from the previous cycles.

However, when analysing the data arriving sequence of D-TDSP transmission shows that all the nodes have broadcasted the data in a synchronous pattern for every 20 cycle, while in the FAST and CSMA/CA only managed to synchronised 10% and 30% of every 20 cycles respectively. The FAST has the lowest synchronicity as the nodes will continuous to update the firing time even when synchronization is achieved.

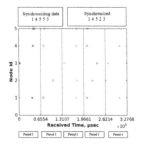 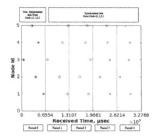 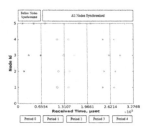

**Fig. 4.** The order of packet received by the basestation from 5 nodes for D-TDSP

**Fig. 5.** The order of packet received by the basestation from 5 nodes for FAST

**Fig. 6.** The order of packet received by the basestation from 5 nodes for random CSMA/CA

## 5.2    Statistical Test on the Synchronization Period for 5 Nodes

In the average synchronization period shown in Table 1, the D-TDSP and the CSMA/CA approach have consistent average period through out the process compare to FAST. This means that the transmission period for the nodes are equally distributed and each node always transmit at the allocated time within the period. The p-value obtained in the T-Test also shown that the transmission period is statistically significant. Hence, the results show that the D-TDSP performs better compared to the FAST synchronization and CSMA/CA and can broadcast in a synchronized and evenly distributed patterns when the numbers of nodes is small.

**Table 1.** Average of synchronization period for 5 nodes.

| Node ID | D-TDSP | | FAST | | Random CSMA/CA | |
|---|---|---|---|---|---|---|
| | Av. cycle period | p-value | Av. cycle period | p-value | Av. cycle period | p-value |
| 1 | 35800.00 | $7.10 \times 10^{-68}$ | 56192.03 | $1.11 \times 10^{-36}$ | 32254.90 | $1.14 \times 10^{-9}$ |
| 2 | 35800.00 | $6.22 \times 10^{-58}$ | 50840.00 | $3.72 \times 10^{-24}$ | 32254.90 | $1.14 \times 10^{-9}$ |
| 3 | 35800.00 | $6.22 \times 10^{-58}$ | 49125.47 | $9.13 \times 10^{-22}$ | 32254.90 | $1.14 \times 10^{-9}$ |
| 4 | 35800.00 | $6.22 \times 10^{-58}$ | 49841.18 | $1.27 \times 10^{-22}$ | 32254.90 | $1.14 \times 10^{-9}$ |
| 5 | 35800.00 | $6.22 \times 10^{-58}$ | 49771.47 | $2.87 \times 10^{-23}$ | 32254.90 | $1.14 \times 10^{-9}$ |

## 5.3 Sequencing of Packet Delivered for 10 Nodes

The packet arrival sequences for 10 nodes transmitting in the networks is shown in Fig. 7, Fig. 8 and Fig. 9.

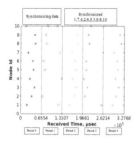 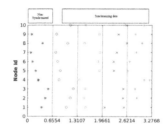 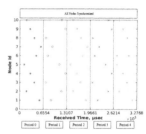

**Fig. 7.** The order of packet received by the basestation from 10 nodes for D-TDSP

**Fig. 8.** The order of packet received by the basestation from 10 nodes for FAST

**Fig. 9.** The order of packet received by the basestation from 10 nodes random CSMA/CA

The results show that the D-TDSP allows each node transmitted in a synchronized and evenly distributed as the packets received are always in ordered. As for FAST, packets transmitted by all the nodes are received at the basestation but not in evenly distributed manners. This is because the nodes in the network were trying to align their time in order to collect the data simultaneously. The D-TDSP has achieved 100% synchronicity for every cycles throughout the transmission while FAST only achieves 10% synchronicity and CSMA/CA 70%. This means that data arrival schedule transmitted by the nodes in the network is not always the same for FAST.

## 5.4 Statistical Test on the Synchronization Period for 10 Nodes

In the statistical test shown in Table 2, the synchronization period shows that D-TDSP and the CSMA/CA have a consistent average cycle period at 34700.00 μs and 32063.34 µs respectively as the p-value is ≤ than 0.01. The consistent average period indicates the nodes in the networks always transmit at the allocated synchronized time. FOR CSMA/CA, the transmission time is configured in the program while for D-TDSP, each node will determine its own transmission based on its neighboring firing.

**Table 2.** Average of synchronization period 10 nodes.

| Node ID | D-TDSP | | FAST | | Random CSMA/CA | |
|---|---|---|---|---|---|---|
| | Av. cycle period | p-value | Av. cycle period | p-value | Av. cycle period | p-value |
| 1 | 34700.00 | $3.35 \times 10^{-226}$ | 27387.62 | $8.96 \times 10^{-22}$ | 32063.34 | $9.35 \times 10^{-11}$ |
| 2 | 33800.00 | $1.15 \times 10^{-209}$ | 34278.92 | $1.12 \times 10^{-22}$ | 32063.34 | $9.35 \times 10^{-11}$ |
| 3 | 34700.00 | $1.12 \times 10^{-221}$ | 34278.92 | $1.12 \times 10^{-22}$ | 32063.34 | $9.35 \times 10^{-11}$ |
| 4 | 34700.00 | $3.92 \times 10^{-227}$ | 34278.92 | $1.12 \times 10^{-22}$ | 32063.34 | $9.35 \times 10^{-11}$ |
| 5 | 34700.00 | $4.00 \times 10^{-234}$ | 33344.77 | $8.89 \times 10^{-22}$ | 32063.34 | $9.35 \times 10^{-11}$ |
| 6 | 34700.00 | $3.95 \times 10^{-289}$ | 34095.28 | $7.82 \times 10^{-22}$ | 32063.34 | $9.35 \times 10^{-11}$ |
| 7 | 34700.00 | $3.08 \times 10^{-221}$ | 34233.08 | $6.80 \times 10^{-18}$ | 32063.34 | $9.35 \times 10^{-11}$ |
| 8 | 34700.00 | $4.46 \times 10^{-209}$ | 33997.90 | $4.63 \times 10^{-24}$ | 32063.34 | $9.35 \times 10^{-11}$ |
| 9 | 34400.00 | $9.45 \times 10^{-226}$ | 33366.90 | $1.55 \times 10^{-21}$ | 32063.34 | $9.35 \times 10^{-11}$ |
| 10 | 34100.00 | $9.37 \times 10^{-230}$ | 34069.78 | $2.39 \times 10^{-19}$ | 32063.34 | $9.35 \times 10^{-11}$ |

### 5.5   Sequencing of Packet Delivered for 15 Nodes

In Fig. 10, Fig. 11 and Fig. 12 below show the synchronization process of the three synchronizations, the D-TDSP, FAST and CSMA/CA.

As the network size is increased to 15 nodes, D-TDSP has managed to broadcast the data to the basestation in an evenly distributed period of time. The D-TDSP had achieved 65% synchronicity. As for the FAST and CSMA/CA, they only managed to maintain 15% and 45% synchronicity respectively. This is due to the increase of interference between nodes during transmission. It is shown that the D-TDSP can avoid interference once the network has been synchronised.

### 5.6   Statistical Test on the Synchronization Period for 15 Nodes

When the number of nodes increases to 15, the average transmission period for each node is not consistent for every cycle in D-TDSP as shown in Table 3. This was because of the large scale of the nodes which can cause delay in transmission from the nodes, the signal period propagated between 32000.00 µs and 34700.00 µs. However, the difference in transmission cycle between the nodes is small compared to FAST which is between 32409.70 µs and 35682.48 µs. The p-value of ≤0.01 also shows that the transmission period for every cycles is statistically significant. This means that the nodes always transmit at the allocated time.

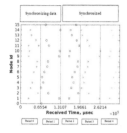
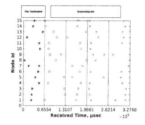
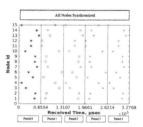

**Fig. 10.** The order of packet received by the basestation from 15 nodes using D-TDSP

**Fig. 11.** The order of packet received by the basestation from 15 nodes using FAST

**Fig. 12.** The order of packet received by the basestation from 15 nodes using random CSMA/CA

**Table 3.** Average of synchronization period for 15 nodes.

| Node ID | D-TDSP | | FAST | | Random CSMA/CA | |
|---|---|---|---|---|---|---|
| | Av. cycle period | p-value | Av. cycle period | p-value | Av. cycle period | p-value |
| 1 | 33900.00 | $6.16 \times 10^{-214}$ | 33722.83 | $1.10 \times 10^{-74}$ | 32212.30 | $1.09 \times 10^{-5}$ |
| 2 | 33900.00 | $9.05 \times 10^{-203}$ | 35095.05 | $8.44 \times 10^{-82}$ | 32745.67 | $7.40 \times 10^{-5}$ |
| 3 | 34200.00 | $1.52 \times 10^{-205}$ | 35095.05 | $8.44 \times 10^{-82}$ | 31998.87 | $4.15 \times 10^{-10}$ |
| 4 | 33800.00 | $3.23 \times 10^{-197}$ | 35095.05 | $8.44 \times 10^{-82}$ | 32105.40 | $1.10 \times 10^{-5}$ |
| 5 | 34700.00 | $4.00 \times 10^{-234}$ | 32273.12 | $4.57 \times 10^{-86}$ | 31998.30 | $1.15 \times 10^{-9}$ |
| 6 | 32000.00 | $9.35 \times 10^{-178}$ | 35173.33 | $1.38 \times 10^{-78}$ | 31999.47 | $5.16 \times 10^{-10}$ |
| 7 | 34200.00 | $1.04 \times 10^{-200}$ | 32409.70 | $1.44 \times 10^{-76}$ | 31998.30 | $1.01 \times 10^{-9}$ |
| 8 | 34200.00 | $2.64 \times 10^{-281}$ | 33988.58 | $7.14 \times 10^{-85}$ | 31999.50 | $1.54 \times 10^{-5}$ |
| 9 | 34200.00 | $8.78 \times 10^{303}$ | 35682.48 | $4.59 \times 10^{-83}$ | 31999.40 | $7.12 \times 10^{-10}$ |
| 10 | 33300.00 | $1.87 \times 10^{-208}$ | 35009.18 | $1.96 \times 10^{-78}$ | 32105.63 | $1.10 \times 10^{-5}$ |
| 11 | 34200.00 | $2.50 \times 10^{-207}$ | 34350.10 | $2.76 \times 10^{-84}$ | 32105.40 | $1.12 \times 10^{-5}$ |
| 12 | 33600.00 | $2.44 \times 10^{-201}$ | 34383.87 | $1.88 \times 10^{-82}$ | 32532.77 | $4.30 \times 10^{-5}$ |
| 13 | 34200.00 | $8.22 \times 10^{-285}$ | 34248.22 | $3.32 \times 10^{-78}$ | 31998.63 | $1.53 \times 10^{-9}$ |
| 14 | 34200.00 | $3.18 \times 10^{-290}$ | 34248.22 | $3.32 \times 10^{-78}$ | 31999.23 | $2.08 \times 10^{-9}$ |
| 15 | 33300.00 | $7.87 \times 10^{-194}$ | 34248.22 | $3.32 \times 10^{-78}$ | 31999.17 | $1.50 \times 10^{-9}$ |

### 5.7 Evaluation of Packet Delivery Rate

In term of the PDR, Fig. 13, Fig. 14 and Fig. 15 shows that the D-TDSP had a PDR of between 98.4% and 100%, while random CSMA/CA had a PDR of between 97% and 100%. For all the networks sizes, D-TDSP has managed to maintain the PDR of above 98% and is higher than the FAST and random CSMA/CA (Table 4).

### 5.8 The Scheduling Effect During Network Interference

In the next two section, two different type of interference are introduced to the networks to evaluate the ability of the three algorithms to maintain the synchronicity of the nodes in the WBN. In this section, a node will be temporary

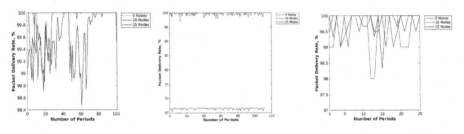

**Fig. 13.** The PDR using D-TDSP    **Fig. 14.** The PDR using FAST    **Fig. 15.** The PDR using random CSMA/CA

**Table 4.** Average of Packet Delivery Rate (PDR) for 100 cycles for 5, 10, and 15 nodes.

| No. of nodes | D-TDSP | | FAST | | Random CSMA/CA | |
|---|---|---|---|---|---|---|
| | Average PDR(%) | p-value | Average PDR(%) | p-value | Average PDR(%) | p-value |
| 5 | 100 | $1.84 \times 10^{-101}$ | 99.71 | $1.62 \times 10^{-222}$ | 99.60 | $1.56 \times 10^{-11}$ |
| 10 | 99.8 | $1.36 \times 10^{-244}$ | 99.75 | $1.03 \times 10^{-274}$ | 99.74 | $2.81 \times 10^{-11}$ |
| 15 | 99.6 | $7.53 \times 10^{-241}$ | 66.50 | $3.93 \times 10^{-267}$ | 99.79 | $1.65 \times 10^{-17}$ |

remove from the network to replicate the node battery replacement. Both experiments will measure and compare the packet arrival sequence in the base station for 5 and 10 nodes.

Figure 16, Fig. 17 and Fig. 18 show the synchronization periods of the D-TDSP, FAST and random CSMA/CA respectively for 5 nodes. It was observed that during the initial time, all of the three techniques shown that all of the nodes were in a synchronized pattern and in-phase. But when a node was added, the sensor nodes in D-TDSP can still maintain its synchronized pattern. While in CSMA/CA, the new nodes managed to transmit during the free slot. However, for FAST, the nodes are not in synchronicity. From the observation, FAST has difficulty in synchronizing the patterns, as the new node will interfere with the other nodes.

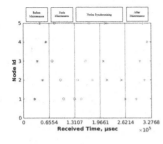
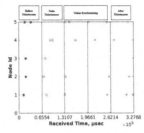
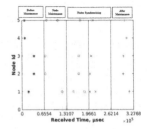

**Fig. 16.** Scheduling process of D-TDSP for 5 nodes when a node is removed temporary    **Fig. 17.** Scheduling process of FAST for 5 nodes when a node is removed temporary    **Fig. 18.** Scheduling process of CSMA/CA for 5 nodes when a node is removed temporary

In Fig. 19, Fig. 20 and Fig. 21, the scheduling effect for 10 nodes are presented.It can be seen that in FAST and D-TDSP, the nodes were able to transmit the data in synchronized patterns. By analysing the synchronicity nodes in every cycles, it is found out that D-TDSP has achieved 100% compared to the CSMA/CA and FAST (50% and 0% respectively). FAST has not been able to maintain the order of the packet received when a failure occurs.

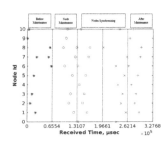
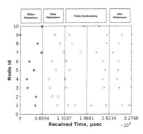
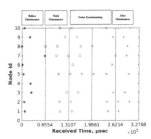

**Fig. 19.** Scheduling process of D-TDSP for 10 nodes when a node is removed temporary

**Fig. 20.** Scheduling process of FAST for 10 nodes when a node is removed temporary

**Fig. 21.** Scheduling process of CSMA/CA for 10 nodes when a node is removed temporary

## 5.9 The Scheduling Effect During Node Addition

In this section, a new node will be added to the networks to evaluate the ability of the WBNs algorithms to maintain synchronicity. The new node introduced will cause the others nodes to hear the broadcast of the packet. The previous node and the next node to transmit will need to adjust its transmission time without affecting the order of node transmission.

The results from Fig. 22, Fig. 23 and Fig. 24 shows the synchronization process when a node added to the network with 5 nodes. From observations, the CSMA/CA has managed to maintained the transmission pattern while in FAST, only 30% of the nodes were in synchronicity after node added. However, in D-TDSP, it shown that the nodes were 100% synchronized after a node added. It can be seen from Fig. 22 that some of the node had delayed their transmission because of the synchronization error.

In the next set of results shown in Fig. 25, Fig. 26 and Fig. 27, the number of nodes in the networks is increased to 10 sensor nodes.

In this scenario, the D-TDSP and CSMA/CA show the nodes are transmitting in synchronizing pattern to the basestation compared to FAST. In D-TDSP, during the synchronization process, some of the nodes were seen transmitted twice in a period. This is because the synchronization convergence time was low. This will cause the nodes time to drift quickly and prompting the continuous resynchronization.

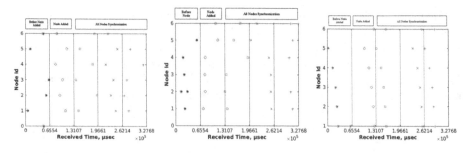

**Fig. 22.** Scheduling process of D-TDSP for 5 nodes when a node is added

**Fig. 23.** Scheduling process of FAST for 5 nodes when a node is added

**Fig. 24.** Scheduling process of CSMA/CA for 5 nodes when a node is added

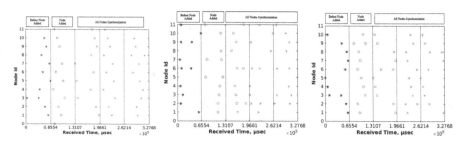

**Fig. 25.** Scheduling process of D-TDSP for 10 nodes when a node is added

**Fig. 26.** Scheduling process of FAST for 10 nodes when a node is added

**Fig. 27.** Scheduling process of CSMA/CD for 10 nodes when a node is added

## 6 Discussion

From the results, it shown that D-TDSP has achieved the highest PDR compared to FAST and random CSMA/CA. As the number of sensor nodes increases, the D-TDSP can maintain the synchronicity of the data. It also shows that during node failure, D-TDSP can manage to transmit the packets in a synchronized period and patterns.

Similarly, when a node was added to the networks, D-TDSP is able to tolerate to temporary radio interference. Hence, any changes of the WBNs the D-TDSP will be able to recover and continue to broadcast the data to the basestation.

## 7 Conclusion

The results above shows that the proposed frog inspired algorithm, D-TDSP, has performed better than CSMA/CA and FAST. The results proved that when a node needed for maintenance, the D-TDSP managed to synchronize the packet data in a short time. Similarly, when there was addition of sensor nodes in the network, the algorithm can readjust its transmission interval. The D-TDSP is able to synchronize the packet sequence and equally distributed the broadcast time of the sensor nodes and is tolerate to failure.

# References

1. Ashraf, D., Aboul Ella, H.: Wearable and implantable wireless sensor network solutions for healthcare monitoring. Sensors **11**(6), 5561–5595 (2011)
2. Campana, J., Gmelin, M., Schoechlin, J., Bolz, A.: Xml-based synchronization of mobile medical devices. Biomed. Eng. **47**, 857–9 (2002)
3. Dhruv, S., et al.: Wearable sensors for monitoring the physiological and biochemical profile of the athlete. Biomed. Eng. **47**, 857–9 (2002)
4. Ikkyu, A., Daichi, K., Yasuharu, H., Masayuki, M.: Mathematical modelling and application of frog choruses as an autonomous distributed communication system. R. Soc. Open Sci. **6**, 181117 (2019)
5. King, R.C., Villeneuve, E., White, R.J., Sherratt, R.S., Holderbaum, W., Harwin, W.S.: Application of data fusion techniques and technologies for wearable health monitoring. Med. Eng. Phys. **42**, 1–12 (2017)
6. Lim, T.H., Lau, H.K., Timmis, J., Bate, I.: Immune-inspired self healing in wireless sensor networks. In: Coello Coello, C.A., Greensmith, J., Krasnogor, N., Liò, P., Nicosia, G., Pavone, M. (eds.) ICARIS 2012. LNCS, vol. 7597, pp. 42–56. Springer, Heidelberg (2012). https://doi.org/10.1007/978-3-642-33757-4_4
7. Maik, P., Steffen, M., Timo, T., Matthias, G., Reinhold, O.: Multi-modal signal acquisition using a synchronized wireless body sensor network in geriatric patients. Biomed. Eng. **61**(1), 57–68 (2016)
8. Monton, E., et al.: Body area network for wireless patient monitoring. IET Commun. **2**(2), 215–222 (2008)
9. Volmer, A., Orglmeister, R.: Wireless body sensor network for low-power motion-tolerant synchronized vital sign measurement. In: Annual International Conference of the IEEE Engineering in Medicine and Biology Society, pp. 3422–3425 (2008)
10. Wang, L., Lou, Z., Jiang, K., Shen, G.: Bio-multifunctional smart wearable sensors for medical devices. Adv. Intell. Syst. **1**(5), 1900040 (2019)
11. Werner-Allen, G., Tewari, G., Patel, A., Welsh, M., Nagpal, R.: Firefly-inspired sensor network synchronicity with realistic radio effects. In: Proceedings of the 3rd International Conference on Embedded Networked Sensor Systems, pp. 142–153 (2005)
12. Yildirim, K.S., Gurcan, O.: Efficient time synchronization in a wireless sensor network by adaptive value tracking. IEEE Trans. Wirel. Commun. **13**(7), 3650–3664 (2014)

# Cybersecurity Analysis for a Remote Drug Dosing and Adherence Monitoring System

Dino Mustefa[1,2(✉)] [ID] and Sasikumar Punnekkat[2] [ID]

[1] Embedded Systems, ALTEN Sweden AB, Stockholm, Sweden
dino.mustefa@mdh.se
[2] Mälardalen University, Västerås, Sweden
sasikumar.punnekkat@mdh.se
https://www.alten.se, https://www.mdh.se

**Abstract.** Remote health monitoring and medication systems are becoming prevalent owing to the advances in sensing and connectivity technologies as well as the social and economical demands due to high health care costs as well as low availability of skilled health care providers. The significance of such devices and coordination are also highlighted in the context of recent pandemic outbreaks underlying the need for physical distancing as well as even lock-downs globally. Though such devices bring forth large scale benefits, being the safety critical nature of such applications, one has to be vigilant regarding the potential risk factors. Apart from the device and application level faults, ensuring the secure operation becomes paramount due to increased network connectivity of these systems and services. In this paper, we present a systematic approach for identification of cyber threats and vulnerabilities and how to mitigate them in the context of remote medication and monitoring devices. We specifically elaborate our approach and present the results using a case study of an electronic medication device.

**Keywords:** Medical IoT · Cybersecurity · Safety · Remote eHealth solutions · Medicine dosage · Remote adherence monitoring

## 1 Introduction

Advanced communication technologies are already an integral part of health services. As smart devices grow in number and equipped with advanced emerging communication technologies, they will be able to communicate directly (device-to-device) and to cloud based health services (device-to-cloud) via either a base station or a gateway. They will form the medical internet of things (MIoT) and will provide diagnostic data access to remotely located disease management system over the internet. This will enable patient mobility and remote medication capabilities as well as continuous adherence monitoring among other interesting

© ICST Institute for Computer Sciences, Social Informatics and Telecommunications Engineering 2021
Published by Springer Nature Switzerland AG 2021. All Rights Reserved
R. Goleva et al. (Eds.): HealthyIoT 2020, LNICST 360, pp. 162–178, 2021.
https://doi.org/10.1007/978-3-030-69963-5_12

applications and possibilities. Though this will bring interesting applications into the medical domain, there is also a great risk that these devices become vulnerable to cybersecurity attacks by adversaries as they are connected to the internet which in turn can put the safety of patients in danger.

Safety practices in critical solutions in the domain are well established and prescribed by safety standards[1]. These standards state clearly how systems should be developed, verified and maintained to minimize risks of accidents and failure over the lifetime of a product. Yet, established safety practices fall short of addressing the new cybersecurity threats and system vulnerabilities that can originate from the growing connectivity and addition of new smart communication technologies and grid components. There are no standards yet on how to deal against these inevitable cybersecurity threats and device vulnerabilities to adversary attacks, but there are guideline documents[2,3] that provide recommendation on what to consider and which controls to implement to reduce the risks and to guard patients from any potential danger. For wider adoption of these devices and their enhanced communication features, it is necessary to do cybersecurity related risk assessment and to mitigation the risks in order to guarantee dependability of health services so that users can rely on them.

The goal of this research is to help creating trustworthy remote medication monitoring system involving intelligent oral medicine dosing device. We have proposed an approach for a detailed cybersecurity threat identification, analysis and mitigation. Following that, we have performed a detailed study on identifying potential threats and vulnerabilities in the system. The investigation covers all system components and scenario including cybersecurity related risks during hardware (HW) and software (SW) design and development (production flow of the HW and SW), distribution (packaging and transportation to end customer), maintenance and post-distribution phases of the product. We have also investigated all network related cybesecurity threats. Finally, we performed an investigation on how cybersecurity preventive strategies can be improved to guard the device against threats that can exploit vulnerabilities in the device as well as on how the device can continue to function despite the system is exposed to a cyber attack.

The paper is organized as follows. Section 2 provides brief information in remote medication and monitoring solutions in general followed by more elaborated information on remote electronic medication and adherence monitoring devices and finally describes safety and cybersecurity challenges. The method and steps required to do threat identification and analysis will be explained in Sect. 3. Section 4 provides description on the use case device and related safety and security challenges and the proposed approach will be used to do risk

---

[1] EN ISO 14971:2007 Medical device – Application of risk management to medical devices.

[2] FDA, Content of Premarket Submissions for Management of Cybersecurity in Medical Devices, 2018.

[3] FDA, Post market Management of Cybersecurity in Medical Devices, 2016.

identification and analysis followed by possible mitigation solutions for identified critical risks. The conclusion remarks are given in Sect. 5.

## 2    Remote Medication and Adherence Monitoring

According to [9], figure of world population aged 65 and above will be doubled in 2025 relative to the figures in 1990. The European population projection in 2012 [7] shows that this will keep on increasing if life expectancy keeps on growing. The same states that the size of working-age population in some regions of Europe will decline considerably including in health care domain. Altogether can have a great impact on the ratio of patients to health care personnel, which necessitates novel remote health care solutions for medication, monitoring as well as treatment purposes.

Adherence is the degree to which a patient follows medication advice and guidelines. Poor adherence is a significant problem across all medical fields and one of the major causes of illness and of treatment failure, and limits providers' abilities to fulfill their ethical obligation of working to improve patients' health and well-being. Patients with chronic diseases and elders require continuous follow up to make sure that they are taking their prescribed medication properly. When patients do not respond to a certain prescribed medication, it can be difficult to determine whether the lack of response is due to nonadherence or whether the medication itself is not effective. [1] found a 76% discrepancy rate between what medicines patients were prescribed, and what medicines they actually took. Up to 25–50% of patients do not take their treatments as prescribed, threatening their health and well-being [2]. A quantitative review of 50 years of research shows; among patients with some disorders (e.g., schizophrenia, diabetes, asthma), nonadherence is the largest driver of relapse and hospitalization. Moreover, misuse or abuse and redirection of controlled substances is a major health issue, with over 50 000 deaths yearly in the USA[4]. In addition to the financial costs of nonadherence, patients who do not adhere to their medications face other potential serious consequences, including higher rates of complications and death. The cost of additional treatments and hospitalizations from nonadherence is estimated to be billions of dollars annually. Furthermore, clinical trials to assess the safety and efficiency of new drugs necessarily rely on proper medication adherence by study participants to obtain accurate data. Adherence or lack thereof has significant impact on the expected treatment outcomes and a significant cost to healthcare domain and society and leads to unnecessary suffering. Therefore, accurate assessment of medication adherence is both clinically important and challenging to all involved parties in the sector.

Existing and emerging advanced smart sensors and connectivity technologies are core components behind a rapid growth of remote care delivery solutions. There are numerous eHealth devices out in the market where patients can medicate themselves with and report disease symptoms. These devices are equipped with smart sensors and advanced connectivity technologies [3] and can track

---

[4] https://www.drugabuse.g.ov/related-topics/trends-statistics/overdose-death-rates.

medication activities and upload either the diagnostic data or just alerts to a remote central disease management system. This brings great values from personalized medication to remote adherence monitoring. But most importantly brings ability to make improved and fast decision by care givers or smart central disease management system as well as to provide feedback to patients through adjusting dosing size or doing a remote critical medical operations. In a bigger picture these solutions will bring many advantages like saving both time and resources, reduce the time required for diagnosis and treatment and reduce needs for hospitalization and emergency room visits. This will improve survival rate, especially to patients living in rural areas, and reduce health care costs both for patients and the health care organizations.

## 2.1   Remote Electronic Medication Adherence Monitoring

Traditionally, clinicians had to rely on patients' self-reporting of adherence to medications [5]. Studies show that self-reporting is unreliable: Patients may have inaccurate memories of taking their medications or may be embarrassed to admit failure to comply or inability to access (lack of finances, not understanding instructions, memory problems) medications. Scholars have pointed to the need for a more accurate measure of whether and when patients take their medications. Products that incorporate adherence monitoring are already on the market and others are awaiting FDA approval. There are different sorts of them:

1. Electronic medicine dosing device
2. Implanted and wearable body sensors [9]
3. Digital medicine: Proteus developed ingestible sensor[5].

Widely-used Medication Event Monitoring System (MEMS)[6] provides very high standard information about adherence. The electronic pillbox[7] is a simple electronic medication adherence tracking device based on a standards that overcomes some of limitations of previously developed similar products [4]. Proteus Digital Health developed ingestible sensor[8] that emits a weak signal when the medication is ingested and the signal is relayed via a patch worn on the abdomen that links with a smart-phone app and records that the medication was taken. eCare Companion[9] enables patient to enter medical information like blood pressure, etc. and fill answers to questionnaires about their timely health condition. This system communicates with sensor devices such as pulse oximeter, weight scale, blood pressure meter, and medicine dispenser to collect data automatically. Philips claims that they provide security and privacy protection of the patient's data, but do not provide details on mechanisms used.

---

[5] https://www.proteus.com/how-it-works/.

[6] https://www.aardexgroup.com/solution/MEMS-adherence-software/22.

[7] http://www.med-tracker.com/.

[8] https://www.proteus.com/how-it-works/.

[9] https://www.usa.philips.com/healthcare/product/HC453564553051/ecarecompanion-patient-app-your-patients-gateway-to-care.

Although *electronic medication devices* may not provide a direct or a complete evidence of medication ingestion as digital medicine does so, they can still provide enough amount of information related to medication adherence. On another hand, combining existing electronic medicine medication devices with an ingestible sensor or wearable sensors would improve efficiency of adherence report. Otsuka Pharmaceuticals' is working on combining ABILIFY (i.e., aripiprazole, which is currently FDA approved for a range of indications in the treatment of serious mental illnesses) with the Proteus ingestible sensor and uses an app to record patients' ingestion of their medication[10]. The app can also track, if the patient wishes, additional information such as self-reported mood and sleep ratings. What these devices have in common is automated collection of patient information, the ability to share that information with designated others, and the link to medication (ingesting a pill, signaling a dose of insulin).

Patients using electronic medication device can log symptom data or wearable sensors can track the state of disease activity and body response to medication, and link it to a connected system, have great potential to improve decisions making on right medication and right dosing which will enable better overall treatment decisions and better outcomes. In a connected system, these decisions can be made faster and simpler, saving both time and resources. Being able to track dosing and track a digital signal if medications are used outside the normal pattern or if the dispensing device is tampered with would allow healthcare and caregivers to act faster if misuse occur, and this feature in itself will have preventive impact on potential misuse.

### 2.2   Safety and Security Challenges

As MIoT products & solutions are getting cheaper and better, more and more patients will be heavily relying on them. To date, there are few accidents or disasters due to faulty or malicious devices, while as the volume and application space increases, these devices will be more prone to such cybersecurity attacks (imagine what an adversary could do with an access to a celebrity's medication device). If these medical end devices fail to work as advertised, at the least patients may lose trust using the devices and at the most, may endanger their lives. Therefore, it is very important to guarantee safety and security of those device. The proposed approach in this paper focuses on guarding such systems from safety failures due to cyber threats.

**Safety Challenges.** Existing methods of tracking medication adherence are far from being perfect and has many potential issues. Most commonly used pill count methods usually overestimate adherence[11]. Medication Event Monitoring Systems (MEMS)[12] suffer from several drawbacks. First, its cap is difficult to

---

[10] https://www.otsuka-us.com/discover/articles-1033.

[11] https://www.affirmhealth.com/blog/pill-counts-a-tool-for-medication-adherence-and-diversion-reduction.

[12] https://www.aardexgroup.com/solution/MEMS-adherence-software/22.

open with arthritic hands. Second, it does not report adherence in real time, so intervention cannot take place if medication time is missed. Third, it does not accommodate the use of pill boxes for sorting medications into daily doses, as are commonly used by the elderly and when multiple drugs are taken. [6] discusses various causes of performance failures in infusion pumps[13]. These medical devices and solutions will be even more prone to failures due to network congestion and cyber attacks as they are increasingly getting connected to the internet.

**Security Challenges.** Cybersecurity threats (*CST*) are often indicative of weaknesses in the system design and those weaknesses make the system vulnerable to attacks by adversaries. As demonstrated[14], adversaries could forge an erratic signal with radio frequency electromagnetic waves in order to hack the implants inside the body. This false signal could inhibit required stimulation or induce unnecessary shocks in human brain and hence endanger life. This is just one example of medical device that can be hacked. Similarly, all MIoT solution can be hacked and threat vector becomes even larger when things are connected in order to push diagnosis and other data to cloud or health server. Therefore, it is paramount to design a structured approach and methods in order to do a comprehensive cybersecurity identification and analysis.

**Mitigations.** Actively looking for potential issues coming from different dimensions (such as SW defects or bugs, HW faults or failures, cyber attacks and human errors) and analyzing them on a continuous basis is very important, followed by identifying both static and dynamic mitigation strategies to ensure fault/attack tolerant operation of remote health monitoring solutions empowered by advanced communication technologies. Regulators, like the FDA, that approves such adherence monitoring products will also need to develop expertise in evaluating these safety and security issues in order to provide rigorous guidelines. The approach proposed below also considers countermeasures and provided some generic control methods in the use case part for certain type of common vulnerabilities in MIoT applications.

## 3  Approach

Here we propose a top-down, step-by-step approach to investigate and analyze cybersecurity threats and vulnerabilities of a medical device followed by control strategies to mitigate critical risks with higher impacts on safety of target patient. Essentially our approach has three stages viz., cybersecurity threat and vulnerability identification, risk assessment and risk control (see Fig. 1).

---

[13] https://www.fda.gov/medical-devices/general-hospital-devices-and-supplies/
infusion-pumps.
[14] https://www.youtube.com/watch?v=FmFLAlZO6ig.

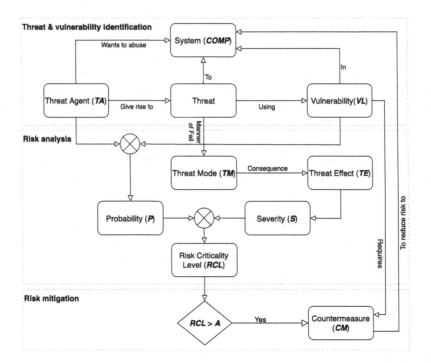

**Fig. 1.** A step-by-step approach to investigate, analyze and mitigate cyber threats.

## 3.1 Threat and Vulnerability Identification

The first stage should focus on identification of cybersecurity threats and vulnerabilities of the system under consideration. This can be done; first by formally describing the different assets or components (*COMP*s) of the system. Threat agents (*TA*s) are people with bad intention and intend to exploit system vulnerabilities to damage the system under consideration. These *TA*s can be different based on the intention they have and all types should be identified. Following that random and intentional cyber threats that can endanger safety of a patient as well as all potential vulnerabilities (*VL*s) in the system should be identified. Both existing and emerging cyber threats should be envisage. Similar systems or products and their threat documentation can be referred to get more existing threats and internal and external information sources can be used to gain a better understanding of potential emerging threats.

## 3.2 Risk Analysis

The risk analysis is guided by the overall risk management process described in[15] (the flow chart is shown in Fig. 2 with minor modification to reflect the

---

[15] ISO 14971: Medical device - Application of risk management to medical devices, 2012.

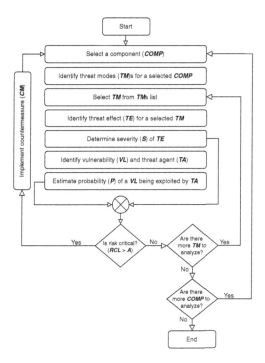

**Fig. 2.** Risk analysis process.

contribution of this paper). According to this standard; failure mode is defined as a manner in which an item fails and failure effect is defined as a consequence of a failure mode in terms of the operation, function or status of the item. A comparable cause-effect chain is suggested in [8] for security threat-effect as threat mode (*TM*) and threat effect (*TE*) and will be used same analogy in our approach as well. Therefore, *TM* is defined as manner of threat impact where as *TE* is defined as consequence of a *TM* in terms of the operation, function or status of the item and both should be identified in this stage.

*TE* is quantified by defining severity (*S*) scale for a system under consideration and typical severity rates are indicated on a scale of 1 to 10 where 1 is lowest severity and 10 is highest. The chances of a *VL* being exploited is quantified by defining probability (*P*) scale and it depends on mainly vulnerabilities in a system but also target environment (*EN*) and the type of *TA* trying to damage the system. Risk criticality level (*RCL*) shows level of damage to a system caused by threat agent. This *RCL* can be determined based on the quantified severity and probability of occurrence. Eventual risk criticality level should be evaluated to know if the risk is minimal or significant. System specific *S*, *P* and *RCL* matrices should all be defined in this stage.

### 3.3  Risk Mitigation

In the third stage of our approach, countermeasures (*CM*s) will be suggested if risk criticality of a threat is not deemed to be acceptable. One or more of the following risk *CM*s can be used in the priority order listed. The first one is to eliminate or reduce risks as far as possible (inherent safety by design), e.g. to add a safety mechanism. The second one is to take protective measures in the medical device itself or in the manufacturing process, e.g. an alarm, in relations to risks that cannot be eliminated as well as information of the residual risk due to any shortcomings of the protection measures adopted (though warning information is not considered as risk control measure, and not intended to lower any risk).

## 4  Use Case

### 4.1  Intelligent Drug Dosing Device

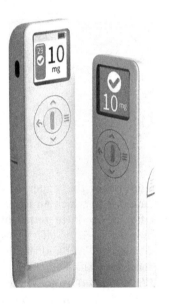

OnDosis, here after called the Device, is a handheld, digital and intelligent medicine container and dosing device to patients with chronic diseases such as attention deficit hyperactivity disorder (ADHD). It will transform existing systems into simpler and more convenient micro particles form integrated to an intelligent device. The Device prototype is shown in Fig. 3 where the display provides status information (e.g., dose size) and a disposable cartridge storing and dispensing a medicine formulated as granules. The device consists of a control unit programmed for a specific medicine and a disposable cartridge containing the specific medicine formulated as granules. The Device will comply in full with the standards[16,17,18,19,20] mandated by Radio Equipment Directive (RED).

**Fig. 3.** The OnDosis drug dosing device

---

[16] EN 55024 Information technology equipment - Immunity characteristics - Limits and methods of measurement.

[17] EN 62479-2010: Assessment of the compliance of low power electronic and electrical equipment with the basic restrictions related to human exposure to electromagnetic fields (10 MHz to 300 GHz).

[18] ETSI EN 301 489-1 ElectroMagnetic Compatibility (EMC) standard for radio equipment and services Part 1: Common technical requirements.

[19] ETSI EN 301 489-17 ElectroMagnetic Compatibility (EMC) standard for radio equipment and services Part 17: Specific conditions for Broadband Data Transmission Systems.

[20] ETSI EN 300 328 Wideband transmission systems; Data transmission equipment operating in the 2,4 GHz ISM band and using wide band modulation techniques.

## 4.2    Closed Loop Medication Management

All dispensing event(s) will be communicated to local monitoring unit (LMU), e.g., a smartphone over a Bluetooth low energy (BLE). Symptoms will be reported using LMU by the patient guided through questionnaires. Physical parameters will be recorded using smart wearable devices attached to a patient and will be communicated to LMU over Wi-Fi. These collected diagnostic data will be used for monitoring the patient condition on local premises using LMU and then will be pushed to cloud for remote monitoring. AI engine

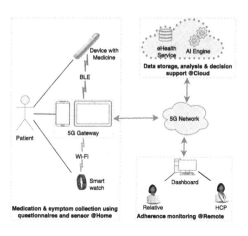

**Fig. 4.** OnDosis connectivity to LMU and Cloud.

will be used for further automatic analysis and remote device setting and hence closed loop medication management (**CLMM**). Figure 4 shows the communication framework and data flows from the Device to LMU and then to cloud. OnDosis connectivity and synchronization of data from device to smartphone application through BLE connection. Further connectivity to health server in order to provide decision support and remote adherence monitoring. This **CLMM** system will enable mobility, frequent & automatic data collection and local & remote adherence monitoring on a continuous basis.

## 4.3    Cybersecurity Analysis of the CLMM System

The approach explained in previous section will be applied in here to investigate cybersecurity related risks of the Device to improve its cyber attack defense to guard safety of patients.

**Threat and Vulnerability Identification.** Brainstorming sessions was performed with the device development team and identified the following details on device assets, usage environments, threat agents, threats and vulnerabilities.

On a higher level, the system comprises the dosing device, network technologies, local monitoring devices & services as well as cloud services as shown in Fig. 4. These different **COMP**s of the system are further listed in Table 1 below.

**Table 1.** Components

| COMP-ID | Components |
|---------|-----------|
| COMP-1 | The Device |
| COMP-2 | Software (SW) storage and SW execution in the Device |
| COMP-3 | Configuration data, event data and device/SW parameters storage |
| COMP-4 | Communications (in the device) |
| COMP-5 | Communications (from device to LMU[a]) |
| COMP-6 | Communication (from LMU to edge/cloud services) |
| COMP-7 | LMU and Diagnostic tools |

[a] Local Monitoring Unit (e.g. Smartphone, Tablet, PC).

The Device is intended for a Home Healthcare Environment in accordance with[21], but can also be used at school or office. The organization, production center and patient's home can be considered as indoor environments where the device will be connected to private network. Where as school, office and public gathering areas are considered as outdoor environments where the device will be connected to public network.

Threat agents can be grouped in different categories based on their intentions as well as target environment. For example, possible thereat agent at indoor environment is insider and intentions can be just curiosity to see certain undisclosed information. On another hand, hacker is a possible agent in outdoor environment and may have intention of harming a patient by altering system settings. Terrorists are agents with way bigger evil intention like mass destruction. Possible types of threat agents are shown in Table 2, but only insider and hacker are considered as threat agent types for the use case system under study.

**Table 2.** Threat agents

| TA-ID | Threat agents |
|-------|---------------|
| TA-1 | Insider |
| TA-2 | Hacker |
| TA-3 | Computer criminals |
| TA-4 | Terrorists |

Table 3 lists threat classes base on STRIDE model. Spoofing consists using someone else credential without their knowledge which usually targets weak authentications. Tampering is modifying a system or a data by adding or removing functional element and destroying or modifying data. Repudiating is hiding

---

[21] IEC 60601-1-11 Medical electrical equipment—Part 1–11: General requirements for basic safety and essential performance.

attacker identity by erasing system logs or acting as some other by stealing credentials. Information disclosure involves data breaching to get a hold of confidential information. Denial of service is preventing user from accessing a system. Escalate privilege is acquiring additional privilege by spoofing user or tampering a system.

**Table 3.** Cybersecurity threats

| CST-ID | Cybersecurity threats |
|--------|----------------------|
| CST-1  | Spoofing             |
| CST-2  | Tampering            |
| CST-3  | Repudiation          |
| CST-4  | Information disclosure |
| CST-5  | Denial of service    |
| CST-6  | Escalate privilege   |

*TA*s abuse a system by using *VL*s in it. For example if a system does not have user identification and authentication, then it is easy for an attacker to do unintended system settings which can result either system damage or death of a patient uses the system. Table 4 lists potential vulnerabilities in a medical devices.

**Table 4.** Potential vulnerabilities

| VL-ID | Vulnerabilities | Description |
|-------|-----------------|-------------|
| VL-1  | Unverified SW   | Poor software verification features |
| VL-2  | Unprotected memory | Poor storage security features |
| VL-3  | Interceptable network | Poor network security features |
| VL-4  | Interruptable network | Poor interference rejection features |
| VL-5  | Unauthorized connection | Poor entity connection verification |
| VL-6  | No user identification | Poor device access authentication |
| VL-7  | Weak user identification | Poor device access authentication |
| VL-8  | Trojan circuit | Poor device electronics protection |
| VL-9  | Weak malware defense | Poor malware protection |
| VL-10 | Unverified data reception | Poor participant verification |
| VL-11 | Unverified entity connection | Poor connection verification |

**Risk Analysis.** According to the approach; threat modes, threat effects, severity of effects, attack probability and risk criticality levels need to be determined in this stage. After surveying and collecting multiple potential threat related characteristics from literature and relevant standards, we zeroed-in on the following aspects based on critical thinking and discussions among development and verification teams.

A threat mode is a manner in which a system fail due to a cyber threat. Adherence monitoring on local device like smartphone will not be available if the BLE channel is continuously jammed. Hence, jamming the BLE network is a *TM*. Table 5 shows list of identified *TM*s for the **CLMM** system and their relation with specific threat type indicated in Table 3.

**Table 5.** Threat modes

| TM-ID | Threat modes | CST-ID |
|-------|-------------|--------|
| TM-1 | Booting from a wrong boot SW | CST-3 |
| TM-2 | Executing a wrong SW | CST-3 |
| TM-3 | Unauthorized SW modification | CST-2 |
| TM-4 | Unauthorized data modification | CST-2 |
| TM-5 | Tampering HW | CST-2 |
| TM-6 | Injecting malware | CST-5 |
| TM-7 | Jamming network | CST-5 |
| TM-8 | Sniffing network | CST-4 |
| TM-9 | Tapping wired connections | CST-4 |
| TM-10 | Repudiating (acting as a genuine sender) | CST-3 |
| TM-11 | Unauthorized access to device features | CST-4 |
| TM-12 | Escalating access right | CST-6 |
| TM-13 | Spoofing (disguise unauthorized changes) | CST-1 |
| TM-14 | Spoofing (stealing credentials) | CST-1 |

Threat effect is a consequence of a certain threat mode. The consequence of jamming the BLE network is interruption of adherence monitoring service, hence the system is no longer available. One or more of the *TM*s shown in Table 5 can result the *TE*s listed in Table 6 and Table 7 shows defined severity scales and their meanings (in the descending order of severity).

**Table 6.** Threat effects

| TE-ID | Threat effects |
| --- | --- |
| TE-1 | Inaccurate functionality |
| TE-2 | Incorrect settings (dose size, time of medication) |
| TE-3 | Incorrect diagnostic data |
| TE-4 | Unable to use the device |
| TE-5 | Wrong cartridge with wrong medicine |
| TE-6 | Adherence service interruption |
| TE-7 | Information disclosure |
| TE-8 | Credential theft |
| TE-9 | Drug abuse |

**Table 7.** Severity

| Level | Category | Description |
| --- | --- | --- |
| 4 | Catastrophic | Patient death |
| 3 | Critical | Permanent impairment or life-threatening injury |
| 2 | Serious | Injury or impairment requiring professional intervention |
| 1 | Minor | Injury or impairment not requiring professional intervention |
| 0 | Negligible | Inconvenience or temporary discomfort |

**Table 8.** Probability of occurrence

| Level | Category | Description |
| --- | --- | --- |
| 4 | Frequent | Likely to happen often |
| 3 | Probable | Likely to occur some times per year |
| 2 | Occasional | Can happen, but not frequently |
| 1 | Improbable | Unlikely to happen, rare, remote |
| 0 | Impossible | Will not happen |

The probability of a system being hacked by a hacker is higher in outdoor than indoor and therefore, target environments should be envisaged when estimating the probability of a vulnerability being exploited. The probability matrix for this system is defined in Table 8.

Table 9 shows defined risk criticality level ($RCL$) matrix which is derived by multiplying the quantified severity and probability of occurrence. If $S$ is serious or below and the probability of occurrence is impossible or below, then the risk is considered as acceptable ($A$). Similarly, if $P$ is improbable or below and the severity is minor and below, then the risk can be again considered as acceptable. Risks which are not insignificant but not clearly unacceptable are considered as

**Table 9.** Risk criticality levels

| | | Probability | | | | |
|---|---|---|---|---|---|---|
| | | 0 | 1 | 2 | 3 | 4 |
| Severity | 0 | – | – | – | – | – |
| | 1 | – | A | A | L | U |
| | 2 | – | A | L | U | U |
| | 3 | – | L | U | U | U |
| | 4 | – | U | U | U | U |

$^A$ Acceptable risk. $^L$ Elevated risk. $^U$ Unacceptable risk.

**Table 10.** Cybersecurity related risks and mitigation

| TMs | TEs | S | VLs | TAs | P | RCL | CMs |
|---|---|---|---|---|---|---|---|
| **The Device** | | | | | | | |
| Unauthorized device access | Drug abuse | 2 | No user identification | Insider | 3 | U | User authentication |
| Unauthorized device access | Incorrect settings | 4 | No user identification | Insider | 3 | U | User authentication |
| Escalating privilege | Incorrect settings | 4 | Weak user identification | Insider | 2 | U | Force strong password |
| **Software Storage and Execution in the Device** | | | | | | | |
| Executing a wrong SW | Inaccurate functionality | 3 | Unverified SW execution | Insider | 1 | L | SW signature |
| Executing a wrong SW | Inaccurate functionality | 3 | Unverified SW execution | Hacker | 2 | U | SW signature |
| Unauthorized SW modification | Inaccurate functionality | 3 | Unprotected memory | Hacker | 2 | U | Memory protection |
| **Configuration Data, Event data and Device/Software Parameters in Local Storage** | | | | | | | |
| Unauthorized data modification | Incorrect settings | 4 | Unprotected memory | Insider | 1 | U | Memory protection |
| Unauthorized data modification | Incorrect settings | 4 | Unprotected memory | Hacker | 2 | U | Memory protection |
| **Communications (in the device)** | | | | | | | |
| Tapping wired connections | Information disclosure | 1 | Trojan circuit | Hacker | 1 | A | |
| **Communications (from device to LMU)** | | | | | | | |
| Spoofing | Incorrect diagnostic data | 4 | Interceptable network | Hacker | 2 | U | Encrypt data on transit |
| Sniffing network | Information disclosure | 1 | Interceptable network | Hacker | 2 | A | |
| Jamming network | Adherence service interruption | 2 | Interruptable network | Hacker | 3 | U | Frequency hopping |
| Repudiating | Incorrect diagnostic data | 4 | Unverified data reception | Hacker | 2 | U | User signature |
| Unauthorized entity connection | Incorrect settings | 4 | Unverified entity connection | Hacker | 3 | U | Entity authentication |
| **Communications (from LMU to edge/cloud services)** | | | | | | | |
| Spoofing | Incorrect diagnostic data | 4 | Interceptable network | Hacker | 2 | U | Encrypt data on transit |
| Sniffing network | Information disclosure | 1 | Interceptable network | Hacker | 2 | A | |
| Jamming network | Adherence service interruption | 2 | Interruptable network | Hacker | 3 | U | Frequency hopping |
| Repudiating | Incorrect diagnostic data | 4 | Unverified data reception | Hacker | 2 | U | User signature |
| Unauthorized entity connection | Incorrect settings | 4 | Unverified entity connection | Hacker | 3 | U | Entity authentication |
| **LMU and Diagnostic tools** | | | | | | | |
| Injecting malware | Unable to use the device | 2 | Weak malware defense | Hacker | 3 | U | Malware protection |
| Unauthorized SW modification | Inaccurate functionality | 3 | Unauthorized access | Hacker | 3 | U | User authentication |

elevated ($L$) risks. Risks in this region may be accepted if further risk is not practicable. Risks critical than elevated region are considered as unacceptable ($U$) risk.

**Risk Mitigation.** Vulnerabilities in a system requires countermeasure in order to reduce cyber related risks. If risk criticality is evaluated as acceptable, shown in green in Table 10, then there is no need for implementation of any countermeasure as the threat impact on safety of a patient is minimal. However, if a threat mode give rise to elevated risk, marked in yellow in the table, or unacceptable risk, marked as red in the table, then the system requires countermeasure implementation to get rid of the corresponding vulnerability. The countermeasure column in the table provides suggestion on generic control mechanisms by leaving specific mechanisms, for example encryption type, for the system developer.

# 5    Concluding Remarks

The result of the use case study demonstrates the impact of cyber threats on today's internet enabled monitoring and medication health solutions. Network and system integration security are important to consider in the product development and need to implement countermeasures for probable cyber related risks to guarantee safety of patients using such products.

A systematic approach is crucial for comprehensive identification of cyber threats and vulnerabilities of the system under consideration. Domain specific cybersecurity standards are prevalent and need to be commercially available to bind product developers to guarantee implementation of necessary countermeasures.

Investigating the security specification of existing advanced communication technologies would be beneficial, as a future work, to select technology with better security implementation and in such a way minimize the effort required from product developers.

**Acknowledgements.** This work is funded by The Knowledge Foundation (KKS), project ARRAY, and by The Swedish Foundation for Strategic Research FiC Project, and the EU Celtic_Plus/Vinnova project, Health5G (Future eHealth powered by 5G).

# References

1. Bedell, S.E., et al.: Discrepancies in the use of medications: their extent and predictors in an outpatient practice. Arch. Intern. Med. **160**(14), 2129–2134 (2000). https://doi.org/10.1001/archinte.160.14.2129
2. DiMatteo, M.R.: Variations in patients' adherence to medical recommendations: a quantitative review of 50 years of research. Med. Care **42**(3), 200–209 (2004). http://www.jstor.org/stable/4640729
3. Fotouhi, H., Causevic, A., Lundqvist, K., Björkman, M.: Communication and security in health monitoring systems - a review. In: COMPSAC 2016: The 40th IEEE Computer Society International Conference on Computers, Software & Applications, June 2016
4. Hayes, T.L., Hunt, J.M., Adami, A., Kaye, J.A.: An electronic pillbox for continuous monitoring of medication adherence. In: 2006 International Conference of the IEEE Engineering in Medicine and Biology Society, pp. 6400–6403 (2006)
5. Klugman, C.M., Dunn, L.B., Schwartz, J., Cohen, I.G.: The ethics of smart pills and self-acting devices: autonomy, truth-telling, and trust at the dawn of digital medicine. Am. J. Bioeth. **18**(9), 38–47 (2018). https://doi.org/10.1080/15265161.2018.1498933
6. Paul, N., Kohno, T., Klonoff, D.C.: A review of the security of insulin pump infusion systems. J. Diab. Sci. Technol. **5**(6), 1557–1562 (2011). https://doi.org/10.1177/193229681100500632
7. Rees, P., van der Gaag, N., de Beer, J., Heins, F.: European regional populations: current trends, future pathways, and policy options. Eur. J. Population/Revue européenne de Démographie 28 (2012). https://doi.org/10.1007/s10680-012-9268-z

8. Schmittner, C., Gruber, T., Puschner, P., Schoitsch, E.: Security application of failure mode and effect analysis (FMEA). In: Bondavalli, A., Di Giandomenico, F. (eds.) SAFECOMP 2014. LNCS, vol. 8666, pp. 310–325. Springer, Cham (2014). https://doi.org/10.1007/978-3-319-10506-2_21

9. Ullah, S., Higgin, H., Siddiqui, M.A., Kwak, K.S.: A study of implanted and wearable body sensor networks. In: Nguyen, N.T., Jo, G.S., Howlett, R.J., Jain, L.C. (eds.) Agent and Multi-Agent Systems: Technologies and Applications, pp. 464–473. Springer, Berlin Heidelberg (2008)

# Author Index

Albertetti, Fabrizio   95

Balogun, Oludolapo D.   20
Balogun, Victor   20
Barbieri, Riccardo   3
Brocanelli, Anna   124

Cecchi, Stefania   35, 124
Chorbev, Ivan   139

Do, Phillip V.   77

Fapanni, Tiziano   55

Garcia, Danson Evan   77
Garcia, Nuno M.   139
Gioacchini, Luca   35

Lameski, Petre   139
Lenatti, Marta   3
Lim, Tiong Hoo   148
Liu, Yi   77
Lopomo, Nicola Francesco   55

Mann, Steve   77
Moreno-Sanchez, Pedro A.   61
Muhammad, Norhafizah   148
Mustefa, Dino   162

Orcioni, Simone   124

Paglialonga, Alessia   3
Pierce, Cayden   77
Pires, Ivan Miguel   139
Poli, Angelica   35, 124
Polo, Edoardo Maria   3
Punnekkat, Sasikumar   162

Rizzotti-Kaddouri, Aïcha   95

Sá, Juliana   139
Sardini, Emilio   55
Sarumi, Oluwafemi A.   20
Sebastião, Raquel   112
Serpelloni, Mauro   55
Simalastar, Alena   95
Spinsante, Susanna   35, 124

Tao, Yi (Summer)   77

van Waterschoot, Toon   3
Villasana, María Vanessa   139

Zanet, Marco   3
Zdravevski, Eftim   139
Zheng, Kai Wen   77

Printed in the United States
By Bookmasters